Why Is My Partner Sexually Addicted?

Why Is My Partner Sexually Addicted?

Insight Women Need

PAUL BECKER, LPC

authorHOUSE®

AuthorHouse™
1663 Liberty Drive
Bloomington, IN 47403
www.authorhouse.com
Phone: 1-800-839-8640

First published by AuthorHouse   02/14/2012

ISBN: 978-1-4685-5011-5 (sc)
ISBN: 978-1-4685-5010-8 (ebk)

Library of Congress Control Number: 2012902082

Printed in the United States of America

Any people depicted in stock imagery provided by Thinkstock are models, and such images are being used for illustrative purposes only.
Certain stock imagery © Thinkstock.

This book is printed on acid-free paper.

Table of Contents

Acknowledgments

To those who shared their stories—and only you know who you are—you will be indispensable to those who will benefit from sharing your journey.

I would like to thank, and acknowledge Cheryl Arenella MD, Patricia Doane, Sherry Hart, and Ann Johnson PhD, who read drafts, and made valuable, and appreciated contributions to this endeavor. I also thank Hilda Schmid who helped with selection of the book cover.

God bless you all.

Other books by Paul Becker, LPC

Letters from Paul
In Search of Recovery: A Christian Man's Guide
In Search of Recovery Workbook: A Christian Man's Guide
In Search of Recovery: Clinical Guide

Dedication

This book is dedicated to all the men and women who struggle to turn sexual addiction into recovery. The Lord blesses all of us—especially those who have yet to find the key to their recovery. Never give up, as the Lord never gives up on any of His creation.

This book is also dedicated to my family. As I age, I realize that relationships with family, friends, and God are at the core of the human experience.

God bless you all.

Introduction

Is this book for me? Why should I read this book?

Women who discover their partner's secret life of sexual behavior:

- Are devastated, outraged, and sad.

- Concerned about their marriage; will it survive?

- Cannot understand how their partner could do this to the family.

- Do not have a working knowledge of sexual addiction.

If you find you agree with any of the above statements, this book was written for you. It is intended to give you:

- An understanding of sexual addiction;

- An understanding of how your partner became sexually addicted;

- An explanation of the devastating nature of pornography;

- An explanation of the role you played in your partner's sexual addiction, if any;

- Insights on how your partner rationalized secret sexual behavior while staying in the marriage bed;

- Insight into what it is like for your partner to live as a sexually addicted person;

- An explanation of the complexity of sexual addiction;

- An appreciation of a new way of life that is part of recovery; and

- A foundation of knowledge to live a recovery journey with your partner.

This book addresses these subjects, and many more. It is intended to help you during these difficult times, and with the decisions you will make about your life and your family.

Is this book just for spouses?

No, if you are:

- A man's significant other, you need answers.

- The mother or grandmother of a sexually addicted man, you too need to know why sexual addiction is part of your family.

- Teenage or adult children; understanding sexual addiction and family dynamics will help you to reject sexual misconduct and help end the pattern of a multi-generational dysfunction.

- Friend; sexual addiction is a huge secret in our communities. The more enlightened friends and fellow travelers are, the greater the prospect is that a sexually addicted man can ask you to be his accountability partner—someone he feels he can trust with his shameful secrets.

- A clergy person; chances are you encounter men who are sexually addicted. You will gain insight on how to counsel both partners in a marriage affected by sexual addiction.

- Therapists and medical doctors; perhaps you are not trained in sexual addiction but you see clients who are dealing with sexual addiction. This book is an excellent resource to give to clients who need information on sexual addiction.

Overview

This book is intended to provide information on the nature of sexual addiction. Woman rarely have a need to understand the origin and consequences of sexual addiction until someone close is found to exhibit sex addiction behaviors. Each of the chapters in this book reveals aspects of sexual addiction, all to help women decide how they will live subsequent to disclosure of their partner's sexual addiction.

Chapter one addresses sexual addiction within the marriage.

Chapter two provides a global insight into the presence of sexual addiction from a clinical perspective. It explores the basics of sexual addiction.

Chapter three presents an insidious underpinning of sexual addiction, namely, shame. Shame fosters secrecy, isolation, and depressed mood, all of which are toxic to healing.

Chapter four explores the roots of sexual addiction, that is, age-inappropriate exposure to sexual material or behaviors and a dysfunctional family of origin.

Chapter five takes a closer look at important coexisting characteristics of sexual addiction, namely, depressed mood, anger, anxiety, and isolation.

Chapter six presents the impact of codependency in a relationship when the male is sexually addicted.

Chapter seven provides information on pornography, an almost universal sex addiction behavior.

Chapter eight presents two stories of lives transformed from sexual addiction to healing.

Chapter nine presents the elements of a healing journey.

Appendix A details multiple sexual behaviors practiced by men.

Appendix B provides an in depth look at the Sex Addiction Cycle and the Acting-Out Ritual.

Appendix C explores the details of how family environment and structure contributes to sexual addiction.

Paul Becker, LPC

Appendix D lists relevant publications in the field of sexual addiction.

Appendix E provides multiple options for counseling and Twelve Step programs.

Note: Men's names associated with each vignettes in the book have been changed to protect their confidentiality. The names in Chapter 9 have not been changed.

**The real act of marriage takes place in the heart,
not in the ballroom or church or synagogue.
It's a choice you make—not just on your wedding day,
but over and over again—and that choice is
reflected in the way you treat your husband or wife.**

Barbara Angelis

Chapter One

Sexual Addiction and Marriage

Choice

Rare is the spouse who is not outraged when she discovers her husband's secret aberrant sexual behavior. Your reaction and emotions may include:

- Confusion, anger, sadness, shame, embarrassment;

- Shattered trust;

- A complete lack of understanding of how your partner could have done this to you and your family;

- Befuddled that he was able to keep the secret so long and how he lived a dual life in your presence;

- Relieved to confirm you are not crazy for suspecting your partner's aberrant behavior;

- Confounded he could engage in acting-out sexual behavior, when, at the same time, he enjoyed the fruits of the marital bed;

- Questioning, "Do I really know this man?"

- Fear of the future—the possibility of living alone, shattered dreams, financial insecurity, loss of friends and community support; and

- Fear you might have contributed to his addiction. (You did not, by definition.)

The reactions women experience upon discovery of their man's sexual secrets could fill many pages. Some women are so outraged that their immediate thoughts are about divorce. However, most women are simply too confused to make a rational decision at the time of discovery.

Ultimately you will have to make a choice as to the position you take in your marriage, whether it is divorce, support, forgiveness, or distancing from your partner.

It is likely your partner is experiencing similar emotions and reactions. For most men who have been discovered, an early reaction is, "how could I have been so stupid?" Another early reaction is fear of losing his family—you and the children. Most men are consumed with shame.

It is not for this author to make a recommendation one way or the other. The solution for each couple may be different. Advice for you includes:

- Don't make hasty decisions. Far too much is at stake.

- Tell your children you and their father are having some difficulties, but neither you nor their father will let the difficulties change the love you and he have for them. Do not use them as sounding boards or a way to punish your partner. Remember children, especially young children, will conclude they played a role in the family's problem and blame themselves. Involving children in the man's sexual addiction problem is a form of abuse in itself. Children cannot be subjected to this trauma.

- Suspend marital relations for an agreed upon period of time. If it is not convenient for your partner to sleep in a different bedroom during this period of time, it may be prudent for him to live outside the home for awhile. Use the time of suspended marital relations to get to know each other better and to form a friendship that is likely absent from your marriage.

- By all means seek counseling for yourself. It is impossible for you to process what is happening in a rational way when you are angry, confused, and in great pain. Of course, therapy is in order for your partner as well. Although it is essential for your partner to obtain counseling, you do not have ultimate control over what he decides to do. You should pursue counseling in any case.

- Join a woman's support group. You may feel very alone in your anger or grief. A support group will give you reassurance you are far from being alone in dealing with your partner's sexual addiction. (Appendix E provides more information on groups for you and your partner.)

- It is prudent for you and your partner to enter marital therapy at some point in the future but, for now, it is critical for your partner to begin to understand the origin and consequences of his addiction and what a recovery journey would look like for him. Marital therapy, in most cases should be postponed for at least six months after the man has begun his therapy.

- Do not manipulate the family bank accounts. While you may wish to protect yourself, until you are in a position where you can make a rational decision about your participation in the marriage, this is not the time to take precipitous action that could leave the family even further wounded. Do obtain copies of bank and investment statements, etc. so, if needed, a base point can be established. However, you may wish to consult an attorney if your partner is using family funds to pay for his addiction.

- If your partner has been arrested for his sexual behavior, don't make any long-term decisions until after the legal proceedings have been completed. Your partner is traumatized at this point and cannot deal with much more on his plate until after the legal proceedings are ended. In cases involving children, the Child Protective Services will determine whether or not your partner should leave the family home.

Perhaps you have questions about your partner's sexual addiction. Here are questions often asked by a spouse when they come in for a joint session.

What was my role in my partner's sexual addiction?

I have never encountered a situation where a wife or significant other caused a male to become sexually addicted. While it is possible for a male to enter sexual addiction as an adult, the overwhelming majority of men who become sexually addicted find the roots of their sexual addiction in their childhood. So, almost certainly, you did not cause your partner's sexual addiction.

Some women still look to themselves for answers to their role in their man's sexual addiction. In his book, *Breaking Free,* Russell Willingham (1999), addresses the spouse's role.

> ". . . [T]he spouse of a sex addict usually assumes that her husband's behavior is a result of some lack on her part. 'If I were only more interested in sex or lost some weight or tried to be more understanding,' she reasons', 'then surely he wouldn't be doing this.'

> What she doesn't understand is that sex addiction is never about the wife, it is about the husband. I'm not saying that she has no influence on her husband's behavior; I'm saying that the issue of sexual brokenness is a lot bigger than that. A genuine sex addict is dealing with issues that predate his wife. Therefore, since she is not the cause, she cannot be the cure.

> Some women resist the idea that their husbands struggle is not their responsibility. They believe that if they could discover the right key to unlock the door, their spouse would come around.

One woman in our group went on a campaign to win back her sexually addicted husband by performing all kinds of sexual exploits. She did everything her husband asked, even subjecting herself to things that were painful and humiliating. After all this, he was still not satisfied. Only then did she realize that it was not in her power to change him."

Can my partner be cured?

Many therapists believe that the word "cured" is misapplied to sexual addiction and all addictions. "Cured" assumes your partner will reach a level of healing which will preclude sexual temptation and any form of sexually acting-out behavior—including sexual thinking or fantasy. While your partner can choose to change his behavior, recovery is a life-long journey. The moment a man believes he is "cured," he is on the precipice of a relapse. The good news is, he can choose to live a life-long commitment to forgo his addictive behavior, but the commitment must be renewed daily.

How long will my partner take to end his acting-out behavior?

Some men are able to end acting-out behavior quickly. However, for many it may take a longer period of time. Each man is unique. Each man came out of childhood with varying degrees of brokenness. Experience has shown a rough correlation between the degree of brokenness your partner experienced during childhood and his ability to give up his dysfunctional behavior. If your partner experienced prolonged and perverse sexual, physical, and emotional abuse, damage is deep; recovery will not be quick. It is not possible to give a definitive answer to this question. Carnes (1991) research and considerable clinical experience postulates thirty specific recovery tasks, including individual and group counseling, working the Twelve Step program, and involving the family in the recovery program. Bradshaw (1988) proposes three stages of recovery. In the first stage, one addresses the primary addiction. In the second, the addict addresses co-dependency, getting in touch with feelings, forgiveness, and working on the inner child. In the third stage, he calls for spiritual awakening and empowerment. Both men agree that recovery is a long process, lasting years.

How will I know when I can trust my partner?

As time goes on, you will get a sense of the progress that your partner is making. Only you have the key to allowing yourself to trust him. Having said that, one change to look for is when you and your children become an ongoing focus of your partner's attention. A sexually addicted man, almost by definition, is totally self-centered. If you see, let's say over a six-month period, your partner's attention to family affairs has significantly changed, perhaps it's time to reciprocate with your trust.

Will my partner slip up on his commitment to sexual sobriety?

There is a difference between one-time or infrequent slips and repetitive slips. A one-time slip means that your partner needs to get right back up on his sobriety horse and continue his ride. Multiple back to back slips require reentering or continuing therapy.

What else needs to be done?

Since partners often lack marital skills, marital therapy is recommended as advised by Carnes and Bradshaw. Since it is unlikely that you and your partner were taught adequate marital skills by your parents, it is never too late for partners to take time to learn.

Often, dating couples begin sexual activity before they have invested in friendship. Once sexual activity begins, the process of getting to know the personhood of the partner ends and their focus becomes one of playing house. The sexual activity needs to be interrupted long enough to give the partners an opportunity to go back and finish the natural part of relationship building—getting to know the soul of the other and building a mutual friendship. Couples therapy may help this process. I recommend finding a therapist who uses the Gottman Theory, "Sound Marital House." I also recommend Imago Therapy.

What can I do to cope with my partner's sexual addiction?

You can help yourself by finding a support group for women who, like you, is struggling with the pain of their man's sexual addiction. It is important for you to reject any shame you feel and to begin to understand your partner has a "cancer" of the soul and only the treatment he chooses to internalize will make a difference. (Appendix E offers multiple group programs for partners of sexually addicted men.)

Other Elements a Spouse Needs to Know about Sex Addiction

For the remainder of this chapter, we will explore other factors at work in your relationship with your partner. They include: codependency, compartmentalization, disclosure, and control. As you read this chapter, see if the descriptions are applicable. Some will apply but some may not.

Codependency

Let me ask you questions about your relationship with your partner:

- At times do you feel you are married to a boy rather than an adult?

- At times do you feel you are the mother in your relationship with your partner?

- Do you have a mental list of characteristics you would like to see your husband change?

- Have you tried to instruct him on how he could make changes in his life?

- Do you find your husband gets upset when you make suggestions or give him advice?

- Do either or both of you tend to avoid dealing with the present moment by using alcohol, drugs, food, sleep or other distractions?

- Does your husband constantly complain about how you keep the house, fix the family food, spend money, or otherwise complain about how you behave?

- Do you find you and your partner each seek to control decisions in your relationship?

- When you are away from your partner, does he complain or get angry about the amount of time you are away?

- Do you wish that your relationship with your partner could be more intimate in a non-sexual way?

- Does your partner lack close male friends?

- Is your partner sexually addicted to you? (Demands sex beyond reasonable expectations?)

If you found you answered yes to at least half of these questions, chances are you are in a codependent relationship with your partner. The next chapter is dedicated to exploring codependency as it affects marriage of couples where the male is sexually addicted.

Compartmentalization

It is difficult for a woman to understand how a man can sexually act out while, at the same time, participate in a marital relationship. A woman clearly sees that sexually acting out in any form is an assault on the marriage bond. She sees acting-out behavior as incredibly selfish. She simply cannot understand how the two behaviors, acting out and marital relationships, can exist side by side.

The answer lies in understanding compartmentalization. A man sees his world as containing multiple boxes. In one box he places his marital relationship, in another box he houses his job, in another box he places his friends and pastime activities, and in the last box he hides his sexual addiction. For him, all the boxes are independent and none touch each other. He does not see how his sexual addiction could impact his job. He may not see how acting out could be an affront to his wife. His sexually addictive behavior began many years before his relationship with you. By the time he married, he convinced himself his sexually acting-out behaviors would go away once he married. He was wrong. It just doesn't happen that way.

A woman, on the other hand, understands the elements her partner puts in his boxes, but for her, all the subjects are lodged in one box. She sees very clearly that when her partner seeks intimacy outside the marriage bed, he takes intimacy away from the marriage bed. To her it could not be any clearer.

How women see the world is correct. During his recovery journey the blessed man will see the world as she does. He will understand that intimacy outside the marriage bed will work to destroy the marriage relationship. Yes, the subject matter in each box is interrelated.

Disclosure

Invariably questions about disclosure of the man's acting-out behavior arise. It is likely, because you are reading this book, you already know some or your partner's story. You may not know it all—and maybe you don't need to at this time—or ever.

Some therapists believe that a fundamental principle of sexual healing is total honesty and openness in the marriage. They argue, unless disclosure is complete, secrets remain which will distance the partners.

Other therapists believe, while disclosure is the ideal, at times full disclosure will cause unnecessary pain to the wife or significant other. A sexually addicted man may want to disclose his secrets to his wife or significant other, not for the sake of healing the marriage, but to free himself from the burden of the secret and to purge his conscience. In this type of disclosure the addicted man is disclosing his secrets to reduce his pain, not to establish an honest and intimate relationship.

In a codependent relationship where the wife or significant other takes on the role of the parent and feels that it is her responsibility to fix him, information disclosed may become a weapon for her to wield against him. For instance, Nancy badgered Tim for more detail about his affairs. Each time he gave her information she would scream that he was not telling her everything and she could never trust him again. Disclosure in a codependent relationship often continues an unbalanced relationship and may not be wise until codependency is addressed either in individual counseling or later in marital counseling. Codependency will be more fully explored in the next chapter.

Disclosure about events that occurred prior to the marriage relationship can be helpful in appropriate detail. Even information about the current acting-out behavior needs to be shared in appropriate detail. Some disclosures may require detail but others may not. Sometimes details cause significant pain for the wife or significant other. For example, it is unlikely the wife or significant other needs to know precisely how the masseuse gave her partner oral sex. The fact that he went to a massage parlor should be sufficient information.

Jane insisted on total detail—of everything that happened. Jane's purpose was not to move on with life once she heard the bad news but to stoke her anger, to keep her anger alive. The more gross the details she heard, the greater her disdain grew for her partner. She insisted on carrying the heavy load of anger when she could have opted for forgiveness which dispels anger. Jane became addicted to her anger and needed fuel to feed her addiction.

Disclosure creates images in the head of the wife or significant other that may or may not be accurate. Taking information and creating one's own story that distorts reality is unhealthy and creates undue pain. Disclosure can be both a blessing and a curse.

Disclosure is best undertaken in the presence of a trained therapist who can put boundaries around appropriate detail and share insights from years of experience.

An article entitled, *Surviving Disclosure of Infidelity: Results of an International Survey of 164 Recovering Sex Addicts and Partners* concluded:

- "Disclosure is often a process, not a one-time event. Even in the absence of a relapse, withholding of information is common.

- Initial disclosure usually is most conducive to healing the relationship in the long run when it includes all the major elements of the acting-out behaviors but avoids the 'gory details.'

- Over half the partners threatened to leave after disclosure, but only one quarter of couples actually separated.

- Half the sex addicts reported one or more major slips or relapses, which necessitated additional decisions about disclosure.

- Neither disclosure nor threats to leave prevented relapse.

- With time, 96% of addicts and 93% of partners came to believe that disclosure had been the right thing.

- Partners need support from professionals and peers during the process of disclosure.

- Honesty is a crucial healing characteristic.

- The most helpful tools for coping with the consequences of sexual addiction are counseling and the Twelve Step programs.

- Disclosure, threats to leave, and relapses are parts of the challenge of treating, and recovering from, addictive disorders." (Schnider, Corley, & Irons, 1998)

Control

For the sexually addicted man, childhood was a time when his need for emotional growth was stifled. For example, your partner, as a child, may have been loved for his good behavior, performance in school or sports, and not because he was a child who was entitled to be loved. As a consequence the child was taught he could control his environment by his performance. He learned, if he were a "responsible" child, the possibility of a favorable parental response was greater.

Other consequences of being overly responsible include a focus on being serious, overly self-reliant, unable to trust, and an inability to relax. Paradoxically, one thing he learned he could control is what he did with his own body. He found when he felt sad, put upon, inferior, or did not measure up to parental expectations, he could escape his environment by sexual fantasy and masturbating to achieve euphoria associated with sexual stimulation. He learned, while his environment did not provide the nourishment he needed for emotional growth, he did control an important element of his world that guaranteed good feelings. Continued repetition of good feelings led to a habit and ultimately sexual addiction. Again, paradoxically, he learned he had to be in control in order to manage his environment.

Spouses of sexually addicted men testify to the need for control that their partner demonstrates in the marriage. For example, their partner may want marital relations on his timetable rather than on a loving agreement to celebrate the marriage bed. They want the behavior of individuals in the family to match their standards. They want what they want when they want it. They learn to repeat the same ineffectual behavior of their parents, that is, to love their spouse and children based on performance. They were robbed of good parental role models. As a consequence, not only are they dealing with sexual addiction in adulthood, their role as a spouse and parent may well be as wanting as was their parents.

All of these factors, codependency, disclosure, compartmentalization, and control need to be addressed in therapy—often by both partners.

Don't let life discourage you; everyone who got where he is had to begin where he was.

Richard L. Evans

Chapter Two

Sexual Addiction from a Clinical Perspective

Sex Addicts Anonymous (SAA), a Twelve-Step program similar to that of Alcoholics Anonymous (AA) is a fellowship of men and women who share their experiences, strength, and hope with each other, so they may overcome their sexual addiction and help others recover from sexual addiction or dependency. As a beginning we will use their definition of sexual addiction.

What is sexual addiction?

"Sex Addiction can involve a wide variety of practices. Sometimes an addict has trouble with just one unwanted behavior, sometimes with many. A large number of sex addicts say their unhealthy use of sex has been a progressive process. It may have started with an addiction to masturbation, pornography (either printed or electronic), or a relationship, but over the years progressed to increasingly dangerous behaviors.

The essence of all addiction is the addict's experience of powerlessness over compulsive behavior, which results in their lives becoming unmanageable. The addict is out of control and experiences tremendous shame, pain and self-loathing. The addict may wish to stop—yet repeatedly fails to do so. The unmanageability of an addict's life can be seen in the consequences he suffers: losing relationships, difficulties with work, arrests, financial troubles, a loss of interest in things not sexual, low self-esteem and despair.

Sexual preoccupation takes up tremendous amounts of energy. As the addict's preoccupation grows, a pattern of behavior (or rituals) follows, which usually leads to acting out (for some it is flirting, searching the *net* for pornography, or driving to the park). When the acting out happens, there is a denial of feelings usually followed by despair and shame or a feeling of hopelessness and confusion." (Sex Addicts Anonymous, 2009).

Let's explore several terms from this definition as well as a few additional characteristics of sexual addiction.

Acting out

Throughout this book the term "acting out" is used in place of naming specific sexual behavior. It is used as a category of behaviors practiced by sexually addicted men.

Wide variety of behaviors

Sexual addiction behaviors tend to fall into two broad categories. The first category includes behaviors which are illegal—and fall under the rubric of sexual offenses.

Some examples of illegal sexual behaviors include:

- Sexual harassment;

- Obscene phone calls;

- Prostitution;

- Rape;

- Incest and child molestation;

- Exhibitionism;

- Voyeurism;

- Child pornography;

- Pedophilia;

- Stalking; and

- Professional misconduct.

Examples of other sexual addiction behaviors that are troublesome yet not illegal, include:

- Compulsive searching for sexually stimulating pornographic images on the internet;

- Compulsive masturbation;

- Multiple affairs;

- Frequent use of paper and video pornography;

- Multiple or anonymous partners including unsafe sex;

- Phone sex;

- Use of chat rooms to stimulate sexual thinking, fantasy, and sexual behavior (Cybersex);

- Voyeurism (non-criminal);

- Frequenting strip clubs;

- Sexual massage and lap dancing; and

- Prostitution (Illegal in most states but not considered a sexual offense).

While most sexual offenders are sexually addicted, very few sexually addicted men engage in illegal sexual behaviors.

The above lists are not exhaustive; several other sexual behaviors can become addictive. (See Appendix A for definitions of common sexually addictive behaviors.)

Denial

Accepting, "I am a sexually addicted man," is frightening and has consequences. When a man admits he has a problem, he is saying to himself, "The most pleasurable activity in my life must end." That is not easy. It is quite common for men who enter therapy to deny they have a serious acting-out problem. In fact, the common response is some form of, "How can I have my cake and eat it too?"

Shame plays a pivotal role in denial as well. To the sexually addicted man, living as an alcoholic or a drug addict seems a far better alternative. He may equate sexual addiction with people who are "perverted." It is difficult for the man to accept he is an addict, a sex addict at that.

For the most part, men in denial believe:

- I am just being a man. It is what men do.

- It's not so bad.

- I work hard and deserve some pleasure.

- I can stop it whenever I want—just not right now.

- I have a stronger libido than the average man.

- If I thought I was hurting somebody, I would do something about it.

Our society hypes sex in the movies, on television, the internet, and even at the Super Bowl. Yet, when a man admits his sexual appetites are out of control, that same society looks down on him. Our society seems to say, it is okay for you to go into the candy store but if we catch you eating any of the goodies we will ostracize you. In this environment, how could a man feel safe and admit he has a problem? Denial seems to be the only way out for many men.

Powerlessness over compulsive behavior

All addictions share this same characteristic of powerlessness over compulsive behavior. It means your partner, despite many pledges to the contrary to himself and perhaps others, is unable to reject all temptations to act-out sexually. He may be sexually sober for periods of time, or may be able to avoid certain practices, but finds himself repeating sexual behaviors of choice, even when he would prefer to stop his acting-out behavior.

Vince's story

Vince is a very successful salesman of medical products. His territory covers several northwestern States. He travels from city to city and from hospital to hospital. Vince relishes his job because it allows him to engage in sexual stimulation with no expectation of being caught. His particular fetish is an adult or erotic bookstore where "peep" shows are featured. The "peep" shows foster sexual stimulation followed by masturbation either alone or with another man.

While he knows his line of medical products well, he understands his sales presentation is critical to closing a deal. He finds sexual stimulation, prior to meeting with a client, calms him down and allows him to think straight. He said, "Orgasm reduces my anxiety of meeting with people."

He was working on a new account at a large hospital in South Dakota. He put many hours into presenting the benefits of his products and socializing with his clients. He had an expectation that after his next meeting with hospital administrators, they would decide to move their business to his company. He was very excited. The new business from this hospital would put him over his annual sales quota.

Vince set a meeting with the hospital administrator for three o'clock on Friday afternoon. He spent the morning reviewing data sheets and other material he needed for his presentation. After lunch and before the meeting he took a taxi to an adult bookstore on the other side of town. He engaged in his normal sexual stimulation activities. He noticed another man who showed considerable interest in his activities. After talking with this man, Vince agreed to go to his apartment nearby.

The excitement of the moment fed into a trance-like state and Vince lost track of time. By the time he ended his liaison with his newfound companion, the meeting time at the hospital had passed. He called the hospital Administrator to apologize but the administrator had gone home for the weekend.

Vince gave up significant financial remuneration for the sake of short-term sexual pleasure. Vince was powerless over his compulsive behavior. This is a point that many partners of sex addicts do not understand. While Vince felt shame and remorse for his behavior, it did not stop him from similar behavior in other cities he visited.

The addict experiences tremendous shame, pain, and self-loathing

In the next chapter, the addict's experience of shame will be explored. Shame is a fundamental characteristic shared by sexually addicted men.

You may find it interesting to learn that pain is often a consequence of sexual addiction. You may wonder how a man experiences pain when, in fact, his compulsive behavior is intended to be pleasurable. You may have observed that your partner appears to be reasonably normal in many ways. The reality for the sexually addicted man is that acting out is his way of medicating the pain of his life. Even more paradoxical, your partner may not even realize the extent of his pain because it is how he has lived most of his life. Often it is only in therapy where the man gains insights into his underlying discontent. The sexually addicted man rarely has a clue how to experience joy, happiness, and a fulfilled life.

The man will expend considerable energy to hide his sexual behavior and his pain. Picture your partner's right hand fully extended with his palm forward and his left hand back by his left ear, palm forward. The right hand symbolizes the effort to which he will go to project the image of a well-adjusted, healthy person. Often he will demonstrate over-achievement in his work, involvement in his church, and other facades he believes will make him look good. The reality is his right hand is only a mask that hides the person who he believes is his real self. He believes the real person is the left hand. The left hand symbolizes his self loathing, lack of self-esteem, and profound shame related to his behavior, and other negative thought processes. He believes he is worthless and mired in so much sin there is little or no hope for him. The left hand lives in constant pain and low-level depression. Depressed mood will be addressed in Chapter 4.

Sean's story

Sean was a high-level executive. He rose through the ranks quickly and had major responsibilities. He was well respected by top level management and by his peers. He seemed to have it all. He had a good analytical mind and was able to keep many projects going simultaneously. He had a unique way of keeping his subordinate managers loyal and interested in his game plan.

Those who knew him were shocked when they read in the newspaper that he had been arrested for stalking a young woman. He explained to his therapist that he lived a dual life. While he had done well in business, he attributed his success to luck. On the other hand, he felt he was a total failure as a husband and father. He despised the fact he was unable to resist temptation. He feared he was intrinsically evil and perhaps possessed.

Sean lived in both his right and left-hand worlds. Ultimately he had to face his demons. He had to rebuild his concepts of both his right and left hand.

Both representations of the right and the left hands are exaggerations. The sexually addicted man is neither as good as he would have others believe nor as evil as he believes his left hand symbolizes. The "real" self requires both hands to be congruent. He has to admit his right hand is a mask against showing the world his addiction and pain. And yes, he has to admit to himself that God does not make junk, including himself. Hopefully he will realize that hope is abundant by means of a life-long recovery journey. When both hands are congruent, he is in the position to begin the work which will lead to a healthy lifestyle, to come out of isolation, and to take measures to end his low grade depressed mood.

There is a clinical term that is used to conceptualize the discordance a man experiences when he lives simultaneously in two conflicting mental constructs. When a man feels distress and is uncomfortable with his competing and conflicting thinking, it is called cognitive dissonance. Cognitive dissonance can be resolved by recognizing the stress-induced state and seeking help to address the conflict. Frequently sexually addicted men continue to live with cognitive dissonance because they believe in the underlying premise that they are evil while trying to deceive the world with their "good guy" act. Unfortunately, the cognitive dissonance to which sexually addicted men subscribe fosters living in low-grade depression. As stated above, many sexually addicted men use acting out to self medicate the pain they experience when life is full of negative vibes.

Unmanageability—out of control

Most sexually addicted men have an intellectual understanding of the consequences of their acting-out behavior. However, their intellectual understanding and their behavior often are not in sync. For example, men in counseling express understanding that if they view pornography on a company computer, loss of job and income could result. Nevertheless, many men continue to view pornography on a computer at work. Once they begin to think about the images they expect to see on the internet, they enter into a trance-like state where all consequences are ignored.

Other men intellectually know that pornography and masturbation impact their ability to share intimacy in their marriage. Men often revert to the emotional state that was created when they were first introduced to unwanted sexual behavior or material (e.g., pornography, sexually stimulating videos, etc.) during their childhood. They need to repeat the high they experienced, the arousal connected with first time exposure. Despite their intellectual knowledge, they continue to seek stimulation outside the marriage. They are out of control.

Jeff's story

Jeff reported he spent $60,000 for on-line pornography, massage parlors, and travel to engage in extramarital affairs. He said he knew it was only a matter of time before the financial consequences would take their toll on his business and family. While he hoped he would not get caught, he admitted to the possibility.

Jeff entered therapy at the insistence of his spouse to deal with outbursts of anger in the home. Jeff believed his outbursts were justified. He said, "If only I would get the respect I deserved from my wife and children, my anger would be history!"

During therapy his therapist helped him to see that the underlying reason for his anger was the lack of self-respect he had for himself, related in part to his hidden sexual behavior. He told his therapist he did not want to deal with his sexual behavior, only his anger.

Jeff chose to quit therapy. He continued his angry outbursts in the home and his sexual quests outside the home. Jeff was not ready to deal with his behavior and its consequences.

The lives of sexually addicted men become unmanageable and, in many cases, are tragic.

In search of the Holy Grail

Sexually addicted men are never satisfied with their latest affair, massage, or the intensity of the pornography they found online. Sex and its pursuit simply do not fill the hole in their souls. Men who pursue multiple partners report that they get bored. They find shortcomings in their victim, which they then use to justify terminating the affair. While some men will continue in an affair for several years, and even marry one of their partners, this is not the norm.

Jacob's story

Jacob is a well built and handsome man. As a teenager, both his contemporaries and older women found him sexually attractive. He was never at a loss for a date and sexual gratification. In his late twenties, he saw his other male friends settle down and take on family responsibilities. He envied his friends, since none of his relationships lasted more than six months. He began to date Susan. Susan was different from any of his other conquests. She seemed to understand him and truly care for him. They married. Shortly after the wedding vows were exchanged, Susan became pregnant. Their son was only two months old when she discovered that Jacob had engaged in affairs, one while they were dating, and a second while she was pregnant.

She told Jacob she would leave him unless he entered therapy. During therapy, Jacob talked about the great thrill he experienced during the pursuit of a new conquest. "The conquest is everything for me," he said. "Once I seduce my conquest, I quickly lose interest—no more challenge."

Jacob said he loved Susan, but felt it was unreasonable for her to expect him to give up that which satisfied him most in life. He said, "Life would just not be worth much if I could not pursue women." He talked about finding the perfect woman, the one that would quell his quest. He said, "At one time I felt Susan would be my perfect woman. I was disappointed when Susan did not turn out to meet my expectations." During the time Jacob was in therapy he met another woman from his church who seemed to be interested in him.

Jacob terminated therapy. Susan divorced him.

Neither Jacob nor any other sexually addicted man becomes permanently satisfied in his pursuit of illicit sex. No man finds the Holy Grail in sex.

Sex addiction cycle and rituals

Sexually addicted men have a sex-addiction cycle and use rituals to lay the foundation for acting-out behavior. (This subject is explained more fully in Appendix B.)

A simplified and shortened version of the acting-out cycle is:

Picture a clock:

- At noon (top of the clock) the man experiences an acting-out trigger. For example, one man's trigger is an attack on his integrity or self-worth. If he even perceives a complaint about his work, his perception will trigger a negative reaction and mood in his mind. For another, it is a feeling of depressed mood.

- At fifteen after the hour on our clock, he begins to medicate his negative feelings by escaping reality. For example, he may engage in a sexual fantasy, or think about a past sexual encounter.

- At 30 minutes after the hour on our clock, he begins an acting-out ritual. The acting-out ritual is a set of actions or behaviors that cause mental and physical arousal (e.g., going onto the internet to check e-mail, but ends up viewing pornography). Arousal leads to orgasm.

- At 45 minutes after the hour, he experiences shame, hopelessness, and guilt from having acted out. He may minimize his actions, and promise himself not to repeat his acting-out behavior. However, the transitory guilt passes, and he returns to the top of the clock to sooner or later begin another cycle.

The sexually addicted man may have different triggers that begin his acting-out cycle. He always has multiple rituals. The concept is the same. The major variation is the amount of time between repetitions of his cycle. Some men believe reduced frequency (what was daily is now weekly) represents recovery. While he is making progress, lasting progress means eliminating the acting-out cycle entirely.

Rarely can a man travel the recovery journey unaided. Counseling, particularly group counseling and Twelve Step programs, are most likely to help the man on his recovery journey. (Appendix E provides information of counseling and Twelve Step programs.)

Sexual addiction begins in childhood

No man wakes up on his 21st birthday and makes the decision to become sexually addicted. For nine out of ten men, the roots of sexual addiction are imbedded in childhood. Most adult sexually addicted men report that they were exposed to unwanted sexual material or behavior anywhere from age three to thirteen. Chapter 3 explores the roots of sexual addiction in detail.

Secrets

Sexual addiction always includes secrets and lies. The child's first exposure to unwanted sexual material or behavior usually begins in a secretive environment. In fact, men often report that the secretive environment taught them that sex is exciting when secretive and forbidden. A secretive view of sex may communicate other messages. The boy learns he cannot speak about his sexual experiences in his family environment.

In her book, *The Sexual Healing Journey: A Guide for Survivors of Sexual Abuse,* Wendy Maltz (2001), says it this way:

- "Many survivors say secretive, compulsive sexual activity is the most intense and satisfying experience they know. Fear of getting caught may increase the adrenaline rush, feeling a chemical high is the secret sex. But like taking drugs, this high is a trap. To maintain the affair, the compulsive masturbation, the illegal sexual activity, the survivor has to lie over and over. Viewing sex as secretive can make it feel shameful. 'This must really be bad if I can't talk about it,' a survivor may think. This kind of sex becomes self-destructive.

- A secretive view of sex makes communication about sex impossible. You can't speak about your real sexual feelings and needs. Because of the lack of open communication, survivors may feel the same as they did in the abuse—all alone during sex."

One would think at some point the man would seek help. Experience has taught that nine out of ten men seek therapy only after having their most intimate secret discovered. In fact, some men only come to therapy to get their spouse off their back.

Jim's story

Jim was caught downloading pornography at work. It happened several times and he was suspended from his job. The suspension triggered discovery of his secrets by his wife. He confessed remorse to both his boss and his wife. At his wife's insistence, Jim sought therapy. He acknowledged he probably spent two or three hours a day seeking sexually stimulating images on the internet. Jim had three young children, and his wife threatened, unless he participated in therapy, she would never allow their children to be present with him alone.

Jim continued to harbor his secret. He far from wanted to give up his most cherished friend, his pornography. Jim thought his therapist knew all of the ins and outs of internet pornography. Jim asked his therapist during his second session, how he could continue to download pornography and not get caught. Jim could not bear the thought of giving up his most prized possession—internet pornography.

Jim's employer transferred him to another part of the country and it is not known if he was able to address his addictive behavior.

Unfortunately, Jim is close to the norm. Most men like Jim, who enter therapy, still find it very difficult to give up their secret behavior. A sexually addicted man is encouraged to find an accountability partner with whom he can share his intimate secrets and temptations. Coming out of secrecy is perhaps one of the most difficult tasks he faces. Coming out of secrecy is also the first step in recovery.

Rev. George's story

Reverend George crashed his computer. He thought surely it was a simple fix to restore his crashed computer. He asked a man in his congregation to take a look at the computer to see if he could get it back up and running. The man found Rev. George's computer crashed because of the vast quantity of pornography he had downloaded to his hard drive.

The man discovered Rev. George's biggest secret. Rev. George was petrified that members of his congregation would learn his secret. He did not know where to turn. Ultimately Rev. George chose to commute away from his home city to join a sex addiction therapy group.

Rev. George realized the consequences of not ending his addiction would be the loss of his position and his marriage. In due course, Rev. George shared his deepest secret with his wife. Contrary to his expectations, his wife gave him positive support. He then had the courage to share his secret with an Elder in his church. Again, he was pleasantly surprised that the Elder did not condemn him. To the contrary, the Elder praised Rev. George's decision to seek help.

Rev. George faced one more hurdle to relieve himself of his toxic secrets. He was challenged to share his addiction and struggle with his men's group at his church. When Rev. George is real and human to his flock, he truly is their shepherd. Rev. George reports he has a stronger marriage and is much happier. He reports feeling respected, contrary to his expectations, by his flock for having come down from his pedestal to share his humanness.

Rev. George shared his most shameful secrets. By doing so he trumped his toxic shame.

Lies men tell themselves to justify acting out

Secrets always lead to a cover-up and lies. The sexually addicted man needs to continue to hide his behavior, the use of his time, and, for some, the expenditure of money. In fact, the man becomes so adept at telling lies, the distinction between a lie and the truth becomes indistinguishable.

The propensity to lie often begins in childhood. In short, the child who begins to use sexual material or behavior to medicate the lack of emotional nourishment he receives from his family, suffers from the shame of his behavior. His shame tells him something is wrong with him. His shame fosters his need to hide his behavior and to lie about his use of time or, if he gets caught, to blame another person and profess "it will never happen again." Lying becomes a defense mechanism he uses to hide his shame.

When a child senses something is intrinsically wrong with him as a person, one of his defense mechanisms is to try to convince the world otherwise. For example, a common form of lying for such a child is to exaggerate. The child believes he cannot be loved simply for who he is, so he exaggerates his accomplishments, feelings, and experiences. For the child who will become sexually addicted as an adult, reality is a lie.

As an adult, lying becomes part of his being. Again, frequently the man is unable to distinguish between the lie and reality. His ability to lie, and more importantly his ability to believe his own lies, reaches a pinnacle when his lies justify his acting-out behavior. Frequently heard examples include:

- I don't go on my computer any more other than to check e-mail.

- I have gotten rid of all my porno web sites and paper magazines.

- I don't need an internet blocker; I can handle this.

- I plan to quit as soon as my wife goes on the pill.

- There is no way I'm going to get caught.

- What I do in the privacy of my own bedroom is my own business.

- The reason I act out is because my wife does not need as much sex as I do.

- I am just looking for intellectual stimulation, not sex.

Lying is most egregious when it is destructive to the family. Lying as a cover to continue sexual behavior is hitting bottom.

The wife or a significant other, who has just learned about her partner's acting-out behavior, probably can think back and enumerate times when he was lying. Sadly, lying probably has not ended yet. It takes a fair amount of time in recovery before the man is willing to face the total reality of his secrets and lying. You are right in wanting to trust your partner, but be patient. It will take time.

Multiple addictions

Sexually addicted men frequently have other addictions. Common addictions, in addition to sex, are alcohol, drugs, eating, work, gambling, spending money, and in particular, perfectionism. Perfectionism is the man's attempt to compensate for his lack of self-esteem by performing at a high level on his job. Perfectionism may also influence his expectations of himself, his wife, and his children's performance. These expectations are rarely reasonable.

Alcohol and drugs may be used to facilitate acting out or in response to the shame and guilt of having acted out.

Men who deal with multiple addictions find it is easier to shed non-sexual addictions before shedding sexual ones. The reason is simple; the man is a walking brewery. Unlike the alcoholic, he need not go anywhere outside of his own body to satisfy his craving. Satisfying his craving begins in his head with sexual thoughts. In addition, the high he experiences from orgasm is more powerful than the high from other addictions.

Compare alcohol and drug addiction to sexual addiction

Someone who is "addicted" to sex will demonstrate a similar brain chemistry response as a person dependent on alcohol or drugs with the drug of choice being sex.

Male sexual addiction is a preoccupation with build-up and achieving release in the form of an orgasm. The mind of the sexually addicted man becomes conditioned to filter almost all human actions and images through a sexual prism. For example, the sexually addicted man will ogle women in the office, on the subway, or walking down the street. He focuses on sexually stimulating body parts. While the obvious—breasts, buttocks, and body curves stimulate sexual thoughts, for some men even the curve of an ankle, the length of the neck, and hands, feet, and facial parts are sexually stimulating. A sexually addicted man will open a newspaper or magazine and immediately seek images that stimulate sexual feelings. He lives in a sexually stimulated state for hours each day.

The driving force for an alcohol/drug addict is the need to induce mood alteration through the use of an external-chemical substance. The sexually addicted man uses his own brain chemicals to achieve an orgasmic high. Both use mood alteration to deal with the problems that come with life.

The difference between male and female sexual addiction

For the male, stimulation and orgasm are the goal. The source of stimulation can be quite different for each man, but the sexual triggers lead the man down the path to acting out.

On the other hand, for many women, sexual addiction is based on an idealized concept of relationship and love. The idealization of the relationship often fills the gap of actual experience from childhood, teenage years, or adulthood. While some women are addicted to sexual stimulation by masturbation, many more compulsively seek a "perfect" relationship. In addition, women may engage in one-night stands in an attempt to satiate, paradoxically, the pain of childhood abuse. Again, for many women the intended outcome is something other than orgasm.

Men who engage in frequent extramarital affairs are not really looking for an "ideal" relationship. The end product is to seduce and experience sexual pleasure.

It is difficult for many women to understand the nature of male sexual addiction. Simply, they have no way of connecting experientially or intellectually with being driven to repeat orgasm after orgasm—for nothing more than an endorphin run in the brain.

Sexually addicted Christian men

You might ask, how can a man, who puts his sexual needs first, call himself a Christian? You may wonder how your partner could participate in church services, Bible studies, and even receive communion while thinking about the next time he can search the internet for sexual images; find privacy to masturbate; or engage in chat rooms, massage parlors, or any other sexual behaviors you consider contrary to the marriage contract.

Your questions are valid and may even be shared by your partner. He too questions his relationship with God. He too wonders if his behaviors are paving his road to hell. Almost with certainty, your partner does not have a loving relationship with his God. Your partner may not know what a loving relationship with God even looks like. Men often take the semblance of understanding God from human relationships. For your partner, his relationship with his own father may have poorly molded his image of God.

Ted's story

Ted's father was a strict man. His father spent considerable time away from the family either at work or at a local bar. When his father came home, he was often abusive as a consequence of alcohol. He would yell at Ted's mother. When Ted's father was abusive, it was gospel according to "St. Dad." There were no ifs, ands, or buts in his "Dad's Gospel." What he said was law. His dad judged every member of the family and community according to the tenets of his personal gospel. Ted did not feel close to his father. He pitied his mother. As Ted grew, his image of God took on that of a judgmental and wrathful God. He had no understanding of God's love because he never experienced unconditional love from his father. When Ted realized he had a sexual addiction, he expected God would judge him harshly. He believed he would be punished for all eternity.

Because they are products of dysfunctional families and experience profound shame related to the aura of sexual addiction, many sexually addicted men see God and the world through Ted's eyes. Ted is far from alone. He, and men like him, use the good feelings from sexual stimulation to enforce the belief that they are not loved for the person they are. They learned to deal with all of life's problems by looking for God in all the wrong places. Sexual stimulation has become their God. They have missed the truth.

With near certainty the relationship between a sexually addicted man and his God are lacking. He sees himself as despicable and unlovable. A key milestone for the man is to understand that his image of God is as perverse as his fears of the consequences of his sexual addiction. His image of God is totally contrary to the reality of God's love.

In his book, *Breaking Free,* Russell Willingham (1999), says he never met a sex addict who understands God's grace. As such, changing a sex addict's understanding of God from one of vengeance to one of unconditional love is a huge step forward. The addict has lived his life in the belief that he does not deserve God's love.

Gerard's story

"My image of God was that of a stern Santa Claus who had a big book where He recorded what I had done right and all my failures. The list of good took one page whereas the evil took the rest of the book.

During a religious retreat I began to comprehend how much God loved me even during my darkest moments. I had moved away from God, but God never moved an inch away from me. This was a life-changing understanding for me.

As a consequence of the transformation, I began to understand how I had isolated myself from those I loved because of my addiction. I learned how joyful life could be when I came out of my cave and began to serve others. I began to see I could reflect the rays of love God sent my way onto others. I realized my sexual lust brought no joy, only pain. This is the understanding I craved for years, but was blind to its reality."

This is the journey that sexually addicted men can choose to travel.

Sex addict and sex offender

The predominant behaviors reported by men who voluntarily enter sexual addiction therapy include compulsive scanning of the internet for pornographic images; engaging in masturbation, marital affairs, and phone sex; and frequenting strip bars/lap dancing, and massage parlors. The sexually addicted man, and those close to him, may fear that he will become a sex offender. Rarely do men who practice the above behaviors cross the line into criminal sex offender behaviors.

It is rare for a man who engages in one or more of these behaviors to then abuse children. Most often the behavior the man finds comforting in adulthood is similar to the behavior to which he was introduced as a child. While many children are sexually abused, most do not become abusers of children as adults. On the other hand, men who go to prison for some form of child molestation, often were sexually abused as children. They too, repeat the behavior to which they were first exposed.

In some cases, a sexually addicted man may be tempted to view child pornography. What starts off as curiosity may become compulsive. The interest in child pornography usually starts in childhood with some form of sexual interaction with other children or sexual abuse. Here again, most men who were exposed to childhood sexual interactions with other children do not, as adults, seek child pornography.

Sexually addictive behavior is often progressive in nature both in terms of specific activities and intensity. Sexually addicted men have a need to seek a more rewarding high. For example, a man addicted to pornography will find the images that once stimulated him no longer do the job. He will continue to seek more provocative images. Progression also means greater intensity. For example, the addict may find sexual thinking takes more of his time and, as a consequence, may masturbate progressively more. To repeat, the progression for the sexually addicted man usually does not progress beyond the man's internal standard of sexual behavior, that is, does not cross the line into sexual offender behavior.

It is unlikely that your partner is, or could be, a sex offender, but let us explore the possibility. If you found that your partner abused children, should you divorce him and forever separate him from your family? That is a decision you will have to make. However, let us look beyond his possible incarceration and explore the potential danger he will present to your family upon release from prison and after treatment.

A 1994 Department of Justice study followed 272,111 people who were released from prison in 15 States. Of that number 9,700 were sex offenders of which nearly 4,300 were identified as child molesters. The number represented two thirds of all sex offenders released from state prisons that year (US Department of Justice, 2003).

This study reported recidivism rates, (the percentage of time a former prisoner is rearrested) for **all criminals** as:

- 67.5% were rearrested for a felony or serious misdemeanor within three years.

- 46.9% were reconvicted.

- 25.4% were resentenced to prison for a new crime.

The same Department of Justice study reported that the recidivism rate for **sex offenders** is much less.

The recidivism rate for all sex offenders who within three years of release commit another sex-based crime was 5.3 percent (men who had committed rape or sexual assault).

The recidivism rate for child molesters is lower. The same Department of Justice study found that an estimated 3.3 percent of the 4,300 released child molesters were rearrested for another sex crime against a child within three years.

The State of Virginia conducted three similar studies and found recidivism rates for sex offenders who were arrested for a subsequent sex crime are around 8 percent. The three State of Virginia studies followed a "cohort," that is, all men released from prison during successive three year study periods. (Recidivism in Virginia, 2001, 2003, & 2005)

One of your primary considerations should be: will my husband, upon release from prison or after extensive treatment, pose a substantial threat of harm to my family or neighbors? The statistics tend to support the conclusion that the risk is low.

Why is the recidivism rate for sex offenders low? Several factors are important:

- In most States the post-prison treatment for sex offenders is very effective.

- Sex offender profiles are different from the profiles of criminals in general. Most sex offenders do not have a long history of criminal offenses. They are not people who are in and out of prison many times. Sex offenders are often sent to prison for long periods of incarceration after their first arrest. (US Department of Justice, 2003)

- Sex offenders find prison difficult. The shame heaped on them during their incarceration is a deterrent to returning to prison.

- Most child molesters do not take stock of the consequences of their actions while they are offending. Once they realize that placing their self-interests first had a profound and painful impact on a child's life, most are horrified at what they have done.

It is not the intent of this book to defend sexual offenders. It is to clarify the level of risk that your partner, if he is a sex offender, is to your family, community, and society in general. By definition, every child is entitled to protection against sexual abuse. In recent years, society has done a better job of educating children against improper touch and encouraging children not to keep secrets. Parents have learned that they need to listen to what their child says rather than to discount the veracity of the child. Child Protective Service Agencies are available in all jurisdictions. States give parents information on where sex offenders reside and work in their communities.

Parents also have learned that sexual offenses are perpetrated most often by adults who are trusted by the family. According to the same study by the Bureau of Justice Statistics (2003), where 9,700 sex offenders were tracked, the majority (93%) of molestations of children were not committed by strangers but by people who were known and trusted within or around the family.

This chapter has introduced you to sex addiction from a clinical perspective. Future chapters will explore other characteristics shared by sexually addicted men including the power of shame and the roots or origin of sexual addiction.

Our sickness is between our ears

Source Unknown

Chapter Three

Universal Consequence of Addiction—Shame

Shame

The man and his wife were both naked, and they felt no shame. (Genesis 2:25)

Scripture tells us that God's vision of humanity did not include sexual shame. Adam and Eve before the fall did not see their bodies as objects of desire, but simply part of their loving relationship. After the fall, Adam and Eve were subject to shame.

> The LORD God made garments of skin for Adam and his wife and clothed them. (Genesis 3:21)

And so shame began for all humanity to experience. Shame is a positive attribute—a self-regulating emotion. A sense of shame tells us that our actions or behaviors do not meet personal or societal standards of acceptability. Humanity uses shame as a restraint against offending others. Shame is part of our conscience. Without a strong and morally correct conscience, society would degenerate into chaos. In general then, a sense of shame is healthy and needed.

A nearly universal trait of sexually addicted men is a profound sense of shame. For a sexually addicted man, shame is not a self-regulating emotion. His shame trumps his sense of being, his sense of self-worth, and his judgment of whether or not he is an acceptable member of society. His shame binds him to negative thinking and depressed mood. Not only does he view the world through his shame, he becomes shame. He sees himself as unable to control his appetites, that is, he is unable to manage his thinking and fantasies and unable to regulate his compulsive need to repeat sexual behavior. He experiences shame as "embarrassment, dishonor, disgrace, inadequacy, humiliation, or chagrin." (Broucek, 1991)

Shame and relationships

For the most part, a sexually addicted man's relationships are filtered through his sense of shame. For example, he is often attracted to a woman who he believes is morally superior as his life partner. In contrast, his sense of shame tells him he is morally deficient. His sense of shame tells him that associating with a morally superior partner may help him overcome his sense of deficiency. Paradoxically, he establishes a relationship that is unbalanced. He positions himself as the naughty boy who gives his spouse power to punish and admonish him. Interestingly, when the man lives in the inferior position, it gives him permission to continue to perform like a naughty child and act out. This syndrome is called codependency and chapter 6 is dedicated to providing a comprehensive discussion of codependency where the male is sexually addicted.

Most sexually addicted men grew up in a family in which shame played a distancing factor in the relationships between family members. The distancing factor of shame often translates into abandonment for the children. The father and/or mother are simply not there for their children. The impact of shame often begins before the child had a sense of relationship. Even a pre-verbal child in a shame-based family can sense the lack of emotional warmth—reflective of shame. The most toxic effect of shame is a distancing between the father and the son—the son who will become addicted. Bradshaw (2005) says,

> "When children have shame-based parents, they identify with them. This is the first step in child's internalizing shame."

In general, addicted men are not proud of their addiction. As such, shame is associated with addiction regardless of the type. (More information on the family structure can be found in Appendix C.)

Generational shame

Shame is not a first generational experience for most sexually addicted men. Often, such men come from families with a history of addiction of one type or another. The history of addiction, and thus shame, often goes back many generations. It is common for addicted men to have a father who was, or is, addicted to alcohol, drugs, gambling, eating, work, and frequently sex. For men who abuse children, it is common to learn that one or both of the man's parents were abused as children, and sexual abuse is often a multi-generational fact in the life of the family of origin.

Shame and the man

A man who feels he is terribly flawed usually does not share his innermost feelings. Picture this: John approaches guests at a party and says,

> "Hi, my name is John. I have a habit that I want to share with you. I love to go on the internet and look for women who have . . . (in detail). Once I find images that stimulate my libido, I begin a perverse ritual of sexually acting out by . . . (in detail)."

It just doesn't happen. And if it did, John would not be invited back to the party or any other social engagement. In reality, John would be hard pressed to share his behavior with any other person, including a therapist. His profound sense of shame keeps his private world of sexually acting out behind a mask of respectability. Guests at the party would be more likely to hear about John's involvement with his church, boy scouts, or business pursuits, but not about his sexually acting-out behavior.

> (As you read John's vignette, did you feel a sense of shame? Were you happy that the details were not disclosed? Would you have felt even more shame if John revealed, in detail, how he achieved orgasm? Sexual shame in the United States is pervasive. For the sexually addicted man, shame is compounded. He deals with his own sense of self-disgust in addition to family shame and societal judgments.)

Shame has a significant impact on the marriage. Most men like John also do not voluntarily disclose their sexual acting-out behavior to their spouses. Even in the marriage, they hide behind a mask of respectability. John's spouse likely will not find out about his acting-out behavior unless she inadvertently walks in while he is engaged in pornography or masturbation. Even then, he will erect a defensive wall by saying, "I don't know what got into me—I won't do it again." But he does—time and again.

Compulsivity and unmanageability of addiction create a man, as one addict put it, "dumber than a brick wall." He tells himself, "My wife will not find out about my affairs." He believes he can live multiple lives without being caught. Then, the big surprise happens: he gets tripped up by an event or an unintended situation. Even if his behavior is discovered for the second, third, or fourth time—he remains shocked, and so does his family. For the most part, men enter therapy only after their shameful behavior, their sick souls, have been exposed.

John Bradshaw (2005) describes the impact of shame on the man:

> "Finally, when shame has been completely internalized, nothing about you is okay. You feel flawed and inferior; you have the sense of being a failure. There is no way you can share your inner self because you are an object of contempt to yourself. When you are contemptible to yourself, you are no longer in you. To feel shame is to feel seen in an exposed and diminished way. When you're an object to yourself, you turn your eyes inward, watching and scrutinizing every minute detail of behavior. This internal critical observation is excruciating. It generates a tormenting self consciousness . . . This paralyzing internal monitoring causes withdrawal, passivity and inaction."

It also causes the man to live in a constant state of a low-grade, depressed mood.

Shame and recovery

As long as shame rules the life of a sexually addicted man, sexual healing is slow and torturous. Until the man begins to look shame in the eye—by facing his secrets and the lies he tells to give himself permission to act out, recovery will be an illusion. Rarely can he acknowledge shame without the help of his family, friend, pastor, or therapist. Since a shame-based man is his own object of contempt, the last thing he needs is condemning words and more shame from his family. As a man contemplates recovery, he needs support, not more shame.

Seth and Janet's story

Seth has been in and out of sexual addiction therapy for years. He has not been sexually sober for more than a week or two at a time. Seth works out of his home several days a week. Once his spouse and children leave for work or school in the morning, Seth's sexual temptation becomes very powerful. Seth frequently bends to temptation. After fighting temptation for a while, Seth will go onto the internet, find sexual images of choice, and subsequently masturbate. If Seth leaves the home early in the morning and heads to the library or Starbucks to use their Wi-Fi to do his work, he does not act out.

During group therapy Seth revealed the nature of his internet sexual images of choice. Seth seeks out transvestite dressing and sexual behavior. As a result of probing, Seth remembered several incidents when he was eight-years-old. He and his sister would go into their mother's bedroom and put on her clothing. Seth found his mother's underwear comforting. Seth characterized his mother as distant and not very affectionate. The therapist hypothesized that Seth found dressing in his mother's underwear as a way of obtaining a sense of the intimacy he craved to have with his mother. Seth was not looking for a sexual connection to his mother, but simply normal emotional nourishment. Seth quickly saw the link between what happened in childhood and his sexually acting-out behavior as an adult. He realized, as an adult, he continued to fill the hole in his soul by repeating similar behavior he experienced as a child.

Seth and his therapists talked about how he could make an adult choice to seek legitimate intimacy rather than act out. He noted, while he and his wife had marital relations, he did not feel a sense of intimacy with his wife. He speculated, if he had an intimate relationship with his wife, the dynamics of his cravings would possibly change.

The therapist suggested to Seth that he disclose his story to Janet. His immediate reaction was he could not do so. He said he felt profound shame related to his internet images of choice, and was fearful Janet would reject him and possibly leave him.

So, even when the sexually addicted man sees a clear reason to disclose his behavior, sexual shame makes it a high hurdle.

Shame and trauma

It is common for a woman who has experienced the trauma of physical, emotional or sexual abuse to use the appearance of moral superiority as a mask against the shame from her trauma. As such, when she sees her partner is as flawed as the person or persons who inflicted trauma on her in her earlier life, she often reacts in horror. Trauma breeds shame. She no longer feels safe, since she believes she can no longer trust her husband, as she could not trust those who abused her.

> "Trauma allows 'shame thinking' to blossom from deep roots in culture, religion, family or our childhood past. As children we tend to blame ourselves for things that happen around us, because we are limited in our capacity to think about others being responsible. In a five-year-old's mind if something bad happened, then she or he must have deserved it, therefore the universe makes sense." (Panos)

Wendy Maltz, (2001) says it this way:

> "The abuse shaped the way I came to think about myself sexually. Because I had experienced strong sexual feelings prematurely, in a situation clouded by fear, and without anyone to help me make sense of the experience, I concluded as a child that there must be something terribly wrong with *me*."

Frequently, trauma and shame impact both partners where sexual addiction resides. As such, both partners benefit from their individual counseling. Both partners and the marriage will be strengthened as each does their own work.

But if anyone causes one of these little ones
who believe in me to sin, it would be better
for him to have a large millstone hung
around his neck and to be drowned
in the depths of the sea.

Matthew 18:6

Chapter Four

The Roots of Sexual Addiction

For nine out of ten men who become sexually addicted, the addiction had its beginnings in childhood.

Model one—sexual addiction has its origin in late teen years or early twenties

For one in ten men who become sexually addicted, the addiction had its origin in late teen years or early twenties. These men grew up in a sexually sterile environment. Nothing sexual was ever mentioned or discussed in his home. His parents and the children were always fully clothed, childhood sleep-overs were not allowed, and, in some cases, the child was home schooled. The child was isolated from life's normal educational events that provided for a healthy understanding of sexuality. This environment created a vacuum of sexual information and experience. The vacuum imploded once he left the family environment. When he experienced sexual stimulation for the first time in his late teens or early twenties, it caused his system to go into overload, and, in turn, made sexual stimulation and orgasm exceptionally pleasurable and desirable. Compulsive repetition of the pleasurable experience turned into sex addiction.

Eliza's story

Eliza was raised in a very devout family. His parents believed children should be protected from the evils of society. Their five children were home schooled. They were not permitted to join scouting or sports activities. Eliza remembers childhood as a happy time. However, he did say he wished his father could have joined more family activities, but he didn't because of long hours of work.

Eliza said that during his childhood years, he didn't even know what sex meant. He remembers no discussion of bodily functions or human nature within the family environment. As a teenager, he did not date. The only exposure he had to girls was his two younger sisters. He remembers asking his mother what the word ". . ." meant that he saw written on the wall of a men's room. She dismissed his question by saying that he should not repeat bad words.

At age eighteen, Eliza was sent off to a small, parochial college. When his dorm mates found out he had never seen a *Playboy* magazine, they flooded him with pornography. Eliza said he devoured the magazines, and began to masturbate daily. He felt he could not tell his parents about his sexual discovery. Eliza said, "As time went by my appetite for sexual material grew. I found that I could not stop, even when I wanted too." He finally talked to a clergy person about his sexual activity and was referred to a pastoral counselor.

Abbott's story

Abbott recalled that as a young child he was frequently ill. "My asthma prevented me from playing outdoors much of the year. My mother was fearful of childhood diseases carried by other children, and would not invite playmates into our home. I passed time by reading, viewing television, and playing video games. I became a loner."

In school, Abbott had just a couple friends. These friends were also interested in playing video games. Abbott said that he was afraid of girls, and kept his distance. He said he remembers being teased by several girls because he was shy. He did not date during high school.

"During my late teen years, a new girl moved in next door. She had no drapes on her bedroom window. Each evening, I watched her from my bedroom window. I used binoculars to watch her undress. I found myself sexually stimulated, and I learned to masturbate during my nightly viewing ritual."

At age nineteen, Abbott was arrested for peeping into windows in his neighborhood. As a form of alternative sentencing, he was required to participate in sex offender counseling.

Each of these men was sexually unaware during childhood. It was not until late in their development that they were exposed to sexual stimulation. For each, late exposure to sexual material was traumatic and formed the basis of their sexual addiction.

Model two—sexual addiction begins in childhood

Most men who are sexually addicted as adults were exposed to a "catalytic event" during childhood. (Carnes, 1994) The "catalytic event" was age inappropriate exposure to sexual materials or behavior. The exposure became the foundation of sexual addiction. It occurred at an age when the child was not intellectually or emotionally ready for such an experience. Often, the event was traumatic, shame filled, and resulted in guilt but, at the same time, caused pleasurable physical or psychological arousal. The event occurred in secret and, in almost all cases, the child expected disclosure of the event would cause adverse consequences. A condition in the family of origin led the child to believe it was not safe to go to either parent. If he had shared his experience with his parent(s), ideally, they would have told the child what happened was not his fault. The event would have been normalized and the severe consequences of future addiction avoided.

The following are several vignettes that include the characteristics generally found in the roots of sexually addicted men. They are recorded in detail to allow you to see how destructive age inappropriate exposure to sexual material and behavior can be. Each of the men in these vignettes did not realize they were becoming sexually addicted. They were introduced to sexuality at a time in their life when their human development did not allow them to make informed decisions.

Jimmy's story

Jimmy was an affable boy around the age of ten. Both of Jimmy's parents were very involved in their vocations. Jimmy's father was a workaholic lawyer. Jimmy's mother was a professor at a local college.

The family belonged to a prestigious country club with all the amenities of golf, tennis, swimming, and social events. Jimmy's parents worked during the day. During the summer they dropped Jimmy off at the country club on their way to work. Jimmy's schedule at the county club was filled with lessons. Early in the morning he had a golf lesson, followed by practice on the driving range. Early afternoon he had a tennis lesson. Often on the days when a tennis match did not follow his lesson, he would go swimming with other boys like himself.

Jimmy liked tennis because, as he understood later as an adult, Steve, the tennis pro, paid a lot of attention to him. Jimmy took to spending afternoon hours in the tennis shack with Steve. Steve taught him how to re-string a racket and other useful skills. One day while spending time with Steve, Jimmy said that he wanted to meet up with his friends and go swimming. However, that day Jimmy had forgotten to bring his swim trunks. Steve said he had a pair of swim trunks in the lost and found that probably would fit Jimmy. He suggested Jimmy try on the trunks at the tennis shack to see if they fit him. As he changed, Steve remarked that for a young boy he had a large penis. He asked Jimmy if he ever touched himself in order to make his penis hard. Steve asked him to show him how he did it. Jimmy felt uncomfortable but he did not want to disappoint his friend Steve, and complied with his request.

As the summer went on, Steve found more opportunities to initiate sexual stimulation with Jimmy. He introduced Jimmy to pornography. Jimmy liked the attention that Steve showed to him, and felt that perhaps their secret behavior was Steve's way of showing him how to be a man—at least that was what Steve said. Jimmy never shared his behavior with his parents. It seemed to him that a time when his parents were open to listening just never happened. Jimmy knew something was wrong with what was happening. He was confused over the conflict between the good feelings he experienced and the secrets Steve made him keep.

After the summer, Jimmy and Steve no longer saw each other. Steve moved to a warmer climate. Jimmy continued to masturbate whenever he felt he wanted to repeat the good feelings he first experienced with Steve. Jimmy began to masturbate more frequently.

Jimmy entered therapy in his early thirties to deal with compulsive masturbation and pornography. Jimmy was committed to shed his victim-hood. His recovery journey took several years, and was successful.

Aaron's story

Aaron entered therapy to address sexual behaviors that he found disturbing. In addition, he wanted help to deal with a rather large collection of paper pornography he inherited from his father.

Aaron told his story. "I thought I grew up in a normal family, but perhaps it was not so normal after all. I now know it seemed normal because I had nothing with which to compare my family. I had a stay-at-home mom and a father who was a foreman at a local sheet metal plant. My brother, Jacob, was seven years older and my sister, Rebecca, was two years younger. I was much closer to Rebecca than I was to Jacob.

My father craved his privacy. He would arrive home from work around 6:00 in the evening, and mother had dinner on the table as he walked in the door. I remember we had very little conversation during dinner except about school. My parents insisted each of us talk about what happened at school. If we were critical of a teacher, my father would declare the teacher correct even without knowing all the facts. My mother never crossed my father, but often complained about him to us children when he was not around.

I don't remember my grandmother who died when I was about three. I do remember my grandfather, but not with fond memories. I remember my grandfather always had a new 'aunt' to introduce to the family. The new 'aunts' did not seem to stay with grandfather very long. My grandparents on my mother's side lived in Spain, and I have no memories of them.

After dinner, my father took his newspaper and went to his study on the third floor of our house. Once he entered his study, he closed the door and, for the rest of the evening, he was not to be disturbed behind his closed door. Only mom was allowed to enter the closed door, but only after she knocked and waited for an invitation. I really didn't mind my dad not being around in the evening, because he was sullen most of the time. The only time I remembered him laughing was when he was drinking and playing cards with some of his friends from work. They got together at each other's homes about once a month. Dad usually worked half the day on Saturday. On rare occasions, he would take my older brother and me to a baseball game. But most of the time he worked in the yard during warm months, and in his shop in the basement during colder months. I never remember mom and dad being affectionate to each other in front of the children. I don't even remember them talking about politics, religion, or any other social subject.

One winter day, I came down with a bad cold and mother made me stay home from school. She had some kind of a doctor's appointment that day, and told me to rest on the couch in the living room while she was gone. She said she would return in a few hours.

For a ten-year-old boy, resting on the couch doesn't last very long, even if he has a bad cold. I started thinking about what was behind dad's closed door on the third floor. I knew I was forbidden to go into his room, but my curiosity got the best of me. With trepidation, I opened the door and peered in. I saw a desk, a chair, some bookcases along one wall, and a reading lamp beside the chair. The bookcases seemed to contain books that I never heard of or had little desire to even open. On the other wall was a large closet. I knew full well I should not open that closet, but I did. Dad had constructed shelves in the closet. On the shelves from floor to ceiling were stacks of magazines. Since I had gone this far, I was curious about what kind of magazine my dad found interesting. The first magazine I opened had a foldout page in the middle with a picture of a woman without clothes that showed her private parts. I was disturbed by the picture, but fascinated. I remember my first thought was why would anyone allow someone else to take a picture of their private parts? As I looked through several other magazines, I was surprised by my feelings. It seemed like fireworks were going off in my head, and even more surprising, I found I had an erection. I was totally confused and scared. I simply didn't understand what this was all about.

After dinner that evening, my father went to his study. After a few minutes, my father stormed into the living room and, in a rage, began to yell at me. He knew I had stayed home from school, and my mother was not home part of the day. Much of what he yelled seemed strange, but it was clear he knew I had entered his closet. He called my brother and sister into the room and pulled off all of my clothes. He yelled something like, 'you want sex; I'll give it to you.' He proceeded to beat me until welts formed on my body. I was so embarrassed that my sister saw my private parts. I was even more ashamed when my brother began laughing at me. I wondered how I could have done such an evil thing.

My shame did not end with the beating. My dad said I needed to be cleansed of my sins, and he put me into our bathtub with cold water. I never remember being so cold, sad, and lonely. Finally, my mother put me to bed. I cried myself to sleep that night. I remember the events of that day in detail. They are as clear in my mind as if they happened yesterday. I can even remember that my father was wearing his blue robe as he beat me. I remember my sister crying as she held her blanket.

I never entered dad's room again while he was alive. I don't think I was ever quite the same after that day. The next day my mother opened the Bible and read to me the passage from Genesis about the fall of Adam and Eve in the garden. I remember thinking I must be as evil as Adam and Eve. How could anyone ever love me?

Later in my teen years, pornography entered my life again. Some of my friends had magazines similar to those I found in my dad's closet. I found I experienced similar feelings when I looked at those magazines as I had felt the day I discovered my father's magazines. I also discovered when I got an erection, I could masturbate to orgasm. Whenever I was down, had not done well on a test, or I did poorly on the basketball floor, I could think about the pictures I saw in magazines, and good feelings would return. I spent a lot of time alone and locked up in my own head."

During therapy, Aaron was encouraged to talk to his brother about what it was like for him to grow up in their family. Aaron thought he was the only black sheep in the family. He was grateful to learn that his experience in dad's room and his beating had been similarly experienced by his brother several years before. Jacob told him he had laughed out of embarrassment during Aaron's ordeal. Aaron learned that pornography and masturbation were serious problems for Jacob as well. Since Jacob was the oldest child, he remembered being beaten several times by his enraged father. Aaron learned many things about his family from Jacob of which he had been unaware.

The one subject they both felt a need to explore was generational sexual behavior. They realized their grandfather, father, and they themselves were sexually addicted. Both Aaron and Jacob had young children, and they pledged to one another to stop passing the family curse on from generation to generation.

Aaron and Jacob continued in therapy together. Both addressed the sexual behavior they carried from childhood into adulthood. Aaron enlisted the help of Jacob to dispose of their father's collection of pornographic magazines. (Jacob had refused to take the collection after their father's death.) They joked that they were probably disposing of materials worth thousands of dollars. However, both felt doing anything other than making sure that the magazines did not fall into the hands of another man, had far more value than any money they could reap from selling the collection.

The brothers also opened a dialogue with their sister, Rebecca, and found that she, too, had been damaged by the family environment. The siblings are now close and are joyful that they addressed the "baked cake" of addiction handed down to them from previous generations.

Patrick's story

Patrick grew up in a family where his mother remarried after Patrick's father had abandoned the family when Patrick was a toddler. Patrick remembers meeting his father when he was an adolescent. His father promised to keep in touch with him, and to return during the next holiday season. His father neither kept in touch nor returned. His stepfather, he remembers, tried to be a good father. He was an Elder in the church. However, as Patrick grew older, he began to see discrepancies in his stepfather's behavior between being a loving father and being very selfish. As a child he remembers extended family members frequently coming and going from his home. Their life centered on their church. Patrick remembers being saved and the acceptance that brought in his family. Patrick had one older sister with whom he was not close. He said she seemed to have considerable problems growing up.

Patrick recalls his introduction to sexual behavior when he was around eight-years-old. A cousin frequently slept over at his house. One evening she was assigned to babysit him. Patrick did not feel it particularly strange that she wanted to give him a bath. On the other hand, he does remember, during the bath, she initiated sex play. After the bath she crawled into his bed with him and continued to touch him. Patrick remembers vividly her touching his private parts. He said he did not remember feeling that way before. However, he knew going to bed naked with his cousin would not have occurred if his parents had been home. He remembers wondering why his cousin chose him.

He remembers very clearly his cousin telling him that if he told anyone about what happened, she would blame it all on him, and he would get punished. She told him he was a bad boy for getting an erection. This made Patrick even more confused. How could such good feelings be wrong and entirely his fault? He agreed with his cousin. He indeed was a bad boy. He also agreed, at least he felt, if he told his parents he would be beaten. Patrick was abused by his cousin several more times during his prepubescent years.

When Patrick became a teenager, he became sexually active. He had a very active dating life that resulted in taking sexual liberties as often as he could.

As an adult, Patrick continued to have affairs but found them unsatisfying. He rated each successive conquest, and found none of them measured up to his standard for marriage. Then he met Amy. Amy was different. She told Patrick she did not believe that God blessed sex outside of marriage. She found out about his sexual past history through some members of her church. She confronted Patrick. Patrick felt it was time to deal with his sexual behavior, and entered therapy.

A Review of the Concepts Found in the Vignettes

As you review the above vignettes see if you can identify in each vignette if and when the following characteristics were demonstrated. For the wife or significant other, it is critical to understand that your partner did not make a conscious choice to bring aberrant sexual behavior into his adulthood. While sexually addictive behavior may have real and caustic consequences in the present time, remember your partner was once a victim, like you are today. However, they cannot remain victims. Society and religious mores call them to accept and repair what went wrong, that is, reject living their adult life in the pits of sexual degradation. They are called to enter into a recovery journey. During the recovery journey, they will have the opportunity to heal and look forward to living an addictive behavior free life.

Your reaction to your partner's sexual behavior may also be conditioned upon your own experiences in childhood, teen, or adult years. Men and women often give off unconscious signals. In discussions with couples where the man is sexually addicted, women often disclose they experienced some form of physical, emotional, or sexual abuse during their earlier life. Your reaction to your partner's condition may also be a reaction to how you were hurt as well. This subject will be discussed further in Chapter 6, on codependency.

Characteristic: Experience a catalytic event

Each of the above vignettes demonstrates how exposure to age inappropriate material or behavior can be the catalytic event upon which adult sexual addiction is based. Not all men readily remember their catalytic event. Sexual exploitation of a child is a traumatic event—the memory of which is often repressed. It is a natural defense for some children who experience a traumatic event to mentally detach in the present moment from the abuse.

Some men don't connect the actions of parents or relatives with sexual abuse. For example, Lewis was bathed by his mother who included hand washing of his genitals until age twelve. Lewis came to counseling to address compulsive masturbation without the use of pornography. It took Lewis several months before he connected his mother's actions with his propensity to masturbate. When Lewis realized the connection, he was horrified because he had begun to repeat the same behavior with his young son. It was not on his radar screen that the actions of his mother could be at the root of his sexual addiction.

It may be difficult for your partner to share his catalytic event with you. It is often difficult for men to share their experiences with a trained therapist, let alone someone he fears may not understand, or may leave him. It is good advice to wait until your partner has been in therapy for at least six months to a year before you ask him to share his secrets and, in many cases, the source of profound shame. The best place to disclose secrets is in joint therapy, because the therapist is trained to explain how your partner's behavior fits into a larger picture of life.

Characteristic: Exposure to age-inappropriate material or behavior

A child experiences many embarrassing moments during childhood. Being caught taking ones sister's candy after Halloween may be embarrassing, but it will not have a lasting effect. Being sent to the principal's office for talking in class is not a lasting traumatic event. Yet, sexual events for children often have negative consequences. Such events are a catalyst for sexual addiction. If the event never occurred, it is axiomatic that sexual addiction could not follow. Sexually addicted men, sooner or later, remember their catalytic event(s). The events are always age inappropriate.

Characteristic: Experience arousal

God made the human to experience sexual arousal. God did not make children to experience sexual arousal at the pleasure of an adult or another person more mature in his or her sexual experience or understanding. In therapy, men report that the feeling of arousal they experienced during their catalytic event was greater than any other arousal experience since that time. The cocaine addict experiences his greatest high the first time he is introduced to cocaine. Some cocaine addicts say they spend the rest of their life chasing that high. Since the high experienced by the child during his catalytic event is so powerful, it is not difficult to understand why he would seek to repeat the pleasurable feelings.

For many sexually abused children, life presents many problems, not just the abuse. For these children, repeating the pleasurable experience of arousal becomes a way of self medicating feelings of abandonment, low self-worth, and lack of love in their life. The repetition of the arousal behavior becomes habitual, and thus the root of adult sexual addiction.

Characteristic: Experience feelings of shame

As noted in Chapter 3, shame and sexual addiction go hand-in-hand, and is often passed down from one generation to the next. Physical, emotional, and sexually abused children often come from shame-based families. Shame binds men to addiction.

Characteristic: Experience feelings of guilt

Shame and guilt often go together but they are different. Guilt is knowing that you have violated your own standards, that is, a reaction to having done something for which one has regret. Shame involves knowing you have done something that others would find reprehensible, and feeling about the activity as you would if you were standing on a stage in front of everyone. Shame goes to the core judgment of self—flawed. Guilt may help a man to choose to deal with his aberrant sexual behavior.

Characteristic: Living in a non-nourishing family environment and structure

Each of the men in the vignettes throughout most of this book was a product of a family that was unable to provide the emotional nourishment they needed for healthy developmental growth during childhood. It is almost universal that men who experience a catalytic event, who go on to become sexually addicted, did not have a healthy, supportive relationship with their fathers. While many men also did not have a strong supportive relationship with their mothers, it is the lack of the paternal support that is particularly toxic.

From a societal perspective, fathers are viewed as normal if they provide housing, schooling, food, clothing, and other necessities. They may even attend some of the child's school or sporting events. However, invariably something is missing from the relationship between a child, who subsequently becomes sexually addicted as an adult, and his father. The child did not bond with his father in a healthy way. There are many reasons why the father was unable to bond with his male children. The most common of which is the father did not inherit a functional role model of how to treat his children differently than he was treated. In addition, alcohol, compulsive work habits, drugs, and even sex may cause a barrier to healthy family relationships. The bottom line is that boys with loving and supportive fathers rarely become sexually addicted.

Exceptions exist to "father disconnect" as the root of the boy's lack of emotional nourishment. One exception is when a role reversal is found among the boy's parents. If the mother exhibits strict authoritative control over the family and is distant emotionally while the father is passive and connected with his children, the disconnect between the mother and her male children is toxic and can lead to sexual addiction.

In a small percentage of men, sexual addiction came from another source. For example, Post Traumatic Stress Disorder (PTSD) may cause significant anxiety and depression. Sexual addictive behavior may follow. In addition, psychiatric disorders, including manic-depressive conditions, schizophrenia, personality disorders and substance dependence can be the source of sexual addiction.

(More information on the family environmental structure can be found in Appendix C.)

Age appropriate time to expose children to human sexuality

You may wonder what is an age appropriate time to expose children to human sexuality?

- Every age is appropriate to expose a child to healthy sexuality.

- No age is appropriate to expose a child to an event that causes sexual stimulation.

Exposure to age appropriate education and guidance should begin when the child first is seen exploring his genitals. Parental reaction to sexuality is critical to understanding the difference between abusive and healthy sexuality.

- Distracting a young child who is touching his genitals is more appropriate than slapping the child's hands.

- When a child is caught playing doctor with a similarly aged neighbor child, it is best to explain to the child that God made us wonderfully, but it's important to keep clothes on when playing with other children.

- When mom or dad finds a pornographic magazine hidden under the boy's mattress, it is an opportunity to share guidance about healthy sexuality.

- When a child asks a question about sexuality, parents can answer the child's question in a way that creates a safe and healthy atmosphere, and encourages the child to ask questions as needed. Parents need to provide age appropriate answers and information. (Many books are available to help parents talk to their children about one of God's greatest gifts to humanity—sexuality.)

Exposing children to age appropriate sexual instruction will actually help to preclude sexual addiction. Children who feel their parents are open to talking about sexual matters feel free to go to the parent if something untoward happens. When a parent is able to explain to the child the behavior he experienced caused normal feelings as God intended, and the event was not his or her fault, the event will have far less impact. In fact, if the event is normalized it is not likely to be a catalytic event.

On the other hand, parents (where one of the partners is sexually addicted) have a tendency to avoid discussions of sexuality because of the shame and guilt present in the family structure. It is this type of environment which causes untoward sexual curiosity and experimentation. Any sexually sterile environment is as likely to produce the next generation of sexually addicted men.

The extremes—an excessively sexualized environment or a sterile sexual environment—are fertile ground for sex addiction.

Internet pornography is affecting the minds of younger children at an alarming rate: so much so that some experts expect an epidemic of illicit sexual behavior. Categorically, a family computer must include blocking software to preclude access to pornography. Exposure to internet pornography is never healthy. Just like a parent who would not allow a child to be exposed to a staph infection, a parent cannot allow the child to be exposed to pornography—even if the blocking software precludes adult access.

By reading this and other recommended books, you have become more aware of the destructive nature of age-inappropriate sexual material and activity. A change in your understanding will help you parent your children and, hopefully, preclude your child falling victim to sexual addiction as an adult.

**The chains of habit are generally
too small to be felt until they
are too strong to be broken.**

Samuel Johnson

Chapter Five

Other Characteristics of Sexual Addiction

This chapter explores how depressed mood, isolation, anger, and anxiety play a role in the life of a sexually addicted man. As you read this chapter, ask yourself if the descriptions apply to your partner. Some will, but some may not.

Chronically depressed mood

Let us step back and view your partner in his everyday life. Below is a series of alternative choices to describe your partner. As you read the choices, decide if he is more like "A" or more like "B."

Your partner is:

A. Always smiling
B. Rarely smiles

A. Always looks to spend time with me and the children.
B. More inclined to spend time by himself watching TV, on the computer, or reading.

A. Always has a new joke on his lips
B. Rarely tells a joke.

A. Rarely sulks
B. Spends too much time sulking.

A. Has a lot of close male friends.
B. Has none or few close male friends.

A. Always looks for new and happy activities to do with the family on weekends.
B. Prefers to work around the house, on the lawn, or is involved in his sport activites or hobbies.

A. Enjoys nonsexual intimacy in the marriage.
B. Has no concept of nonsexual intimacy. Intimacy equals sex.

A. Enjoys a lively conversation at the dinner table.
B. Converses but it is rarely lively or enjoyable.

A. Rarely complains.
B. Often complains about work, neighbors, government, church, etc.

A. Is seen as a joyful person.
B. Rarely experiences joy.

If you found your partner resembles more "B's" descriptions than "A's," he may be chronically depressed. "B" descriptions are traits experienced by a man who is chronically depressed. The vast majority of sexually addicted men live in a state of chronically depressed mood.

Living in a chronically depressed state can be traced to several factors:

- Shame may be a characteristic of your partner's family of origin. If so, as a child he bought into shame as a way of living. As an adult, if shame defines him as a person, he will find it difficult to feel good about his life.

- Since your partner, as a child, likely did not receive emotional nourishment he needed to develop healthy feelings about himself, he may withdraw into himself to seek stability. If your partner, as a child, was deprived of love and joy, then, as an adult, he sees what is wrong with life and is blinded to the joys of life.

- When your partner, as a child, formed a habit of sexual stimulation, he confirmed shame in his life. While he found pleasure in sexual stimulation, the pleasure was short lived. Over time his remorseful (shameful) feelings lasted much longer each day.

- Your partner, as a sexually addicted adult, knows that he is different. He believes if he exposes his behavior to public scrutiny, rejection will follow. If his understanding of his bad self prevails over anything positive in his life, the result is he will live in a chronically depressed mood.

The following section explains why a chronically depressed mood contributes to sexually acting-out behavior. And by deduction, it also explains why the sexually addicted man, as part of his recovery journey, must take positive steps to come out his chronically depressed mood.

Dysthymic Disorder

The mental health community calls a chronically depressed mood a *Dysthymic Disorder*. Dysthymia is characterized as a depressed mood lasting at least two years during which time the person experiences a continuous feeling of malaise. (American Psychiatric Association, 2000) Not much in life is going great but, at the same time, one is not so deeply depressed that he cannot function. Perhaps another appropriate descriptive term is *low-grade depression*. Those who experience low-grade depression often have low energy, low self-esteem, and a general feeling of hopelessness.

Perhaps a visual tool will help to explain how low grade depression relates to acting out. This visual tool is called The Addict's Life Scale. This scale ranges from zero to fifty, in ten-point increments. Each benchmark on the scale correlates with a relative mood level. Let's start at the top of the scale and work our way down. The first benchmark on the scale, shown on the following pages, is the fifty-point benchmark. This level signifies the mood associated with acting-out behavior and the feeling of euphoria one feels during the build-up and orgasm. By frequently repeating his acting-out ritual, the addicted man may try to maintain life at the fifty-point benchmark. Let's call this level the "euphoric level."

However, sustaining life at the fifty-point benchmark is difficult because of the shame and guilt that follow acting-out behavior. It becomes a futile chase for the impossible.

One step down, we signify the forty-point benchmark as the normal functioning level. It is the mood level of solid strength and energy. Let's call this level the "Great to be alive" mood level. A recovering addict can see that the margin of difference between the forty-point benchmark and the fifty-point benchmark, his former acting-out behavior level, is only one step, or ten-points away. When he chooses to live at the "Great to be alive" (forty-point) benchmark, he begins to understand that a ten-point gain by acting out is not worth the shame, anger, and discomfort associated with the fifty-point benchmark.

The next step down is the thirty-point benchmark. It is a level below the "Great to be alive" mood level. Let's call this level the "Bad day level." A person who regularly functions at the forty-point benchmark realizes that life has its ups and downs, and it is okay to be down for a short period of time. A person who normally lives at the forty-point benchmark realizes that the thirty-point benchmark is a level he visits, but he does not live there.

The twenty-point benchmark constitutes a low-grade depressed mood or a Dysthymic Disorder level. For most sexually addicted men it is the mood level that accompanies awakening each morning. Life is simply not meeting expectations. One man said, "I got in a rut and I furnished it!" When asked, the sexually addicted man talks about unfulfilled relationships with parents, siblings, and, in particular, his spouse. He has few, if any, close friends. He feels lonely much of the time. He looks for more from life but does not seem to ever find it. He finds he procrastinates because he fears failure.

Profound feelings of shame haunt him. The tone with which he describes himself has elements of "poor me." Other men suffering this low-grade level of depression use the cliché, "Life is a bitch and then you die."

The twenty-point benchmark is a dangerous level. The sexually addicted man sees acting out as an easy way to increase his mood (a thirty-point jump). He will rationalize his acting-out behavior just to "feel better." Men who live at the twenty-point benchmark live in constant low-grade pain. Their underlying discomfort with life is always nagging at their brains. Society teaches us that when we are in pain, we are entitled to take medicine to relieve the pain, and for the addict that medication is acting out sexually.

In this way, the recovering addict who maintains life at a 20 point benchmark is far more susceptible to slipping back into acting-out behavior.

The ten-point benchmark represents full-scale depressed mood. This person finds it difficult to eat, sleep, and to go about daily life. Sexually addicted men rarely experience full-scale depressed mood. They are survivors, and although they do not feel good about themselves, they tend to weather life's daily blows. However, public discovery, particularly when there are legal or divorce implications, is an exception to the survivor mode for the sexually addicted man, and full-scale depression may follow. When the mask comes off, when the deficient self is exposed, friends and relatives often express critical judgments. Those who he once thought would support him often shun the addict most. For the addict's family and acquaintances, the sudden contrast between the person publicly portrayed and the addict's real self is a shocking contradiction that takes time and understanding to resolve.

The zero-point benchmark represents institutionalization. The man who finds himself at the zero-point benchmark is no longer in control of his life. He is not capable of making rational decisions. Other than to identify this level on the scale, it will not be addressed further.

With this introduction, let's look at the Addict's Life Scale.

Addict's Life Scale

50 - Acting-out mood. The feeling of euphoria one feels during the build-up and experience of an orgasm.

40 - Normal Functioning Mood. The ideal mood level of a normally functioning adult. It is the "great to be alive" mood level.

30 - Bad Day Mood. A level to visit but not to stay at.

20 - Low-grade Depressed Mood or Dysthymic Disorder. Where most addicts live life.

10 - Full Scale Depressed Mood. The person barely functions.

0 - Unable to Function Mood. The person is often institutionalized.

The most important element of the Addict's Life Scale is the thirty-point contrast between the twenty-point benchmark, low-grade depressed mood, and the fifty-point benchmark, the acting-out mood. When the addict chooses the fifty-point benchmark, a thirty-point gain, he feels a sense of euphoria, a high, a rush. The orgasm is the end product. It is the goal; it is the relief from life's pain. His pain is so unacceptable he is willing to go for the short-term fix.

He tells himself:

- I need this!

- I can't live without my fix.

- Life is a bear. I deserve this to be happy once in awhile.

- I earned it!

- Oh, the hell with it; I am going for it!

Pete's story

Pete entered therapy because he had been found out. Mary, his wife discovered pornographic images and movies on his computer.

"Mary told me I either seek help, or live in the garage. Not only did I have problems with pornography and masturbation, I worked at least seventy hours a week. I was more married to my job than Mary. I worked long hours, sometimes even weekends. I spent very little time with my teenaged twin boys, Rob and Tom."

Pete, a mortgage broker, quipped, "You have to make hay when the sun shines." Pete had one male friend, a drinking buddy from school. He thought his marriage was acceptable, but he did not think that his wife was his best friend. In fact, he said he did not have a best friend. Since he worked so many hours, he told himself, "Sunday morning is my time to sleep and relax." Pete had not been to church for years. The one thing that Pete did have was a healthy stock portfolio. He mused, "Lot of good that will do me when I die from working too hard!" Pete admitted his life was not what he had hoped it would be.

Pete came to therapy scared. Mary had gone back to work when their boys were out of grade school, and he knew she made enough money to support herself. He said, "I am afraid Mary is so unhappy she might leave me. Who could blame her? If she leaves me, how will I live? Yes, I have treated her very badly, but I need her."

After several months of therapy, Pete was open to making changes in his life. He explained, "I now understand how choosing healthy and uplifting activities could reduce my need to self-medicate my pain. I also know I will be a much happier person if I change my priorities. I need to address my relationships with my family. I need to put them first."

Pete agreed to participate in marriage therapy with Mary. They worked on a marriage plan. He agreed to come home for dinner no later than 6:30 each evening. He and Mary agreed to spend one evening during the week getting to know each other again. They chose to read several books together and to discuss each other's views about what they read. They agreed to do something together each weekend, either a day or evening event. Other changes followed as they became friends.

Pete also addressed his relationship with Rob and Tom. He said, "I am concerned my boys will soon be grown and I will have missed it all. I need to let them know that I take responsibility for my failure to be there for them up to now, and begin to 'walk the talk.'"

Pete sat down and talked to his sons. He told them about his addiction to porn and masturbation and the reasons why, as he understood them. The boys already knew, all too well, about Dad's addiction to his work. He asked them to help him repair the damage he had done to their relationship. His sons loved baseball. They agreed to attend minor league games together. Pete made it a point to make time to be with, and talk to them. His boys were more than happy to get their dad back.

Pete attended a Twelve Step sexual addiction program and made a good friend with whom he began to share his walk. His friend became his accountability partner.

The next important change Pete made was to repair his relationship with his God. He said, "I asked my family to join me Sunday mornings at church. At first, they did not buy in. I guess they, too, liked the family habit of sleeping in on Sunday mornings. That's another bad habit I taught them! As I showed by my actions, I was serious about changing my life; Mary joined me at church each Sunday. One New Year's morning, Rob and Pete said, 'We talked about what kind of New Year's resolution we could make—something meaningful. Dad, we would like to join you and Mom at church each Sunday.'"

Pete made a conscious decision to include activities and other changes that raised his mood functioning to the forty-point benchmark. These activities not only raised Pete's mood and reduced his desire to act out, but they made his life much closer to the life he wanted.

The key for the addict is to choose to change his life so that the forty-point benchmark, the "great to be alive" mood level, becomes the norm rather than the twenty-point benchmark level, low-grade depressed mood. As noted earlier, the differential between the forty and fifty benchmark is only ten points. Men who make the effort to change how they live, so as to experience frequent forty-point benchmark level, "Great to be alive" feelings, find that a ten-point differential is not enough of a reward to offset the negative consequences of acting out.

Because thinking, feelings, behavior, and moods have been ingrained over many years, it is unlikely that many men will find they can live at the forty-point benchmark level most of the time, or even for most of each day. However, to change the power of the addiction, your partner can begin to include mood-lifting behaviors in his daily life. It is possible to consciously choose to move out of one's rut.

Isolation

Closely associated with the chronically depressed mood is living in isolation. Shame, depressed mood, poor self-image, and other feelings of inadequacy lead men to live in isolation as opposed to living a more gregarious existence.

By now you probably can deduce how childhood sexual behavior, a dysfunctional family of origin, and shame led your partner, as a child, to pull into himself—a state where he felt safer. Men, when they are a product of abuse and a dysfunctional family, report that they rarely had many friends growing up. They call themselves loners. With the advent of video games it was much easier to isolate themselves.

As your partner grew into adulthood, he may have ventured out of his cocoon if he went away to school, to the military, or found a job in a different city from his home. In addition, most sexually addicted men tend to come out of their cocoon when drinking alcohol. Alcohol reduces inhibitions. In fact, dating you may have been a way for him to maintain isolation. A one-on-one relationship is more acceptable to him than to pursue an attachment to a larger group of people.

You may or may not feel your partner fits this isolation description. You may wish to ask him what he prefers, and why. Chances are his words will convey he prefers an environment where he is less exposed to people, criticism, controversy, etc. In fact, some sexually addicted men avoid television shows which depict controversy or adverse and difficult relationships. They find arguing, controversy, and people experiencing emotional pain, difficult to watch. You may be the only person with whom he feels he can disagree or argue.

Anger

Pent-up ill feelings about self are a breeding ground for anger. When your partner has a choice to focus on what is going right in his life, as opposed to what's going wrong, he may see the negative side more clearly.

While he may not be fully aware that he sees himself as a victim, he acts like a victim. A victim is angry when he feels he has not been treated fairly. In particular, harking back to the concept of control, your partner may express anger when he senses he has been bested, or lost an argument. When he feels he is no longer in control, as he sees it, he is like a child who wants to throw a temper tantrum. Perhaps, you have seen the five-year-old child come out of your partner and throw a temper tantrum from time to time. Sexually addicted men are often emotionally stunted at the age at which they were abused. When they are stunted at an early age, emotional reactions, even from an adult body, are childlike.

Anger can be expressed as sarcasm, criticism, condescension, yelling, or withdrawal. Your partner may have demonstrated all of these anger characteristics. However, an expression of anger which causes the most difficulty in any relationship is when he simply withdraws and refuses to talk. He simply chooses to end the conversation or argument. He acts like a child who feels he is not winning at his game of marbles, picks up all his marbles, and goes home. Displaying anger by withdrawing is a destructive force to any marriage.

Interestingly, sexually addicted men often display anger while driving. If someone cuts them off, they are outraged. If they are not winning the race, they are distraught. One wife characterized her husband as driving with his penis, his small head rather than the head on his shoulders. For some reason, men feel the road is a battleground for their manhood. God help you, if you criticize his driving.

Me-ism

Sexual abuse is a traumatic event in the life of a young boy. Children ages four or five are self centered, as God intended. It is a time of achieving identity, and as such, the child's focus is directed to mastering his environment. It is a time of occasional temper tantrums intended to convince a parent to give into his wants. If a child who is focused on getting what he wants is traumatized, his emotional development is frozen in time. As an adult he acts very much like a young child. Life is all about satisfying his wants. Life is all about "me."

Children, who are the product of dysfunctional families, for their own protection learn to control their environment. A child who seeks control is internally focused on survival. Survival often looks like turning all emotions and actions inward so as not to be hurt by the dysfunction within the family. If that child is not rescued from his perception of the "terrors of the night," he will grow into adulthood internally focused. He will look like a selfish adult who is overly attuned to getting his "me" needs satisfied. These men, as adults, are often sexually addicted. One of their needs is to avoid the negativity of life by repetitively experiencing the good feeling generated by sexual stimulation.

Situational anxiety

Anxiety is a unique situation for some sexually addicted men. Some men simply do not fall into any of the descriptions of sexual addiction covered so far in this book. And yet, acting-out behavior rules their lives.

Some men feel a constant sexual tension in their bodies. It is almost as if their genitals occupy a sensor lobe in their brain. They are constantly aware of a nagging feeling in the groin that will not go away. The only way to quell this constant and nagging feeling is to masturbate.

Ted's story

Ted is a successful architect. However, whenever he works under a deadline, he experiences considerable difficulty in completing the project. During the day he procrastinates and does just about any other work or task to avoid the project and its deadline. He knows, full well, all he has to do is concentrate and get the job done. Usually the job does not involve applications beyond his technical skill, but he feels others might criticize his work. Ted always carries the possibility of failure in his head, even though he remembers only one time when a colleague criticized his design. The criticism was easily addressed.

The anxiety Ted feels is almost unbearable. His feeling of anxiety seems to lodge in his genital area. The only solution which Ted believes will quell his feeling of genital tension is to masturbate. He said he does not masturbate to enjoy the orgasm, but to get it over with so he can concentrate. Ted masturbates several times a day to reduce his anxiety. He sees orgasm as his only relief to his anxiety.

If your partner sounds like Ted, he needs counseling and medication to address his anxiety. Counseling will help him to deal with his underlying fear of failure and medication will level the playing field to reduce the physical manifestation of tension.

Chronic anxiety

Chronic anxiety, like a chronically depressed mood, is a condition in which some sexually addicted men live day in and day out. Anxiety dominates the man's life and he is in a constant state of unrest or has a continuous feeling of apprehension. Living life is not pleasant. Mack's story, below, illustrates the impact of chronic anxiety.

Mack's story

Mack thought that his nickname was a curse. He said:

"I never felt like macho Mack. My Dad began to call me Mack when I was young. He would say, 'Where is my Mack truck?' I was not a Mack truck, I was Matthew! I grew up feeling like life was going to hand me a bad deal. I constantly felt uneasy and apprehensive. I was sure that, given the opportunity to succeed, I would pluck defeat out of the jaws of victory. Dad thought so too. He constantly told me how much I disappointed him."

Mack was sexually abused by Benjamin, a family member. The abuse continued throughout his childhood years.

"I lived in fear of Benjamin, who told me I had the body and face of a pretty girl. *And they called me Mack?* I felt sad and angry. Why did I have fine features? Was it my fault that Benjamin always found me when no one else was around? I was afraid to tell Mom or Dad about him. I was sure Dad would tan my hide so I could never sit again. To top it all, I began to stutter. Stuttering just seemed to make matters worse for me. School kids taunted me, 'pretty boy—talks like a girl.' I felt ashamed and no good."

Life got even worse for Mack. Around age ten he began to wet the bed at night.

"Dad really yelled at me when he found out I wet the bed one night. He called me a sissy. I had to hide my problem from him. I found a big piece of plastic to put on my bed on top of the sheets. I was able to awake when I felt wet and the problem ended."

But Mack's problems continued.

"In high school, I was a loner and would masturbate frequently, just like Benjamin had taught me. I dropped out of college after my first year. I found a job in a video store. I lost that job because I could not concentrate and was irritable. I came to work late because I had difficulty sleeping. Masturbation was the only fun I had."

Mack was diagnosed with a Generalized Anxiety Disorder, (American Psychiatric Association, 2000) and is in therapy.

Mack's unfortunate life experiences taught him not to trust himself or anyone else. He was totally isolated in his pain and anxiety. He would first have to address his childhood experiences. He would have to internalize that others had hurt him. He had no choice in the events that had shaped him. He would need the guidance of a skilled therapist to help him rethink his life perspective, and to begin to understand that he is a person of worth who could make new choices as an adult. Both his anxiety and masturbation are chronic. Only after Mack is able to see outside the wall he has built to protect himself from pain will he begin to defuse his chronic anxiety.

Patrick Carnes (1991) frames the issue of the effect of sexual abuse:

"Abuse and neglect deepen this distrust of others and further distort reality. Children who are neglected conclude they are not valuable. In addition, they live with a high level of anxiety because no one teaches them common life skills or provides for their basic needs. Children find ways to deaden the anxiety they inevitably feel, and they do so compulsively. For sex addicts, compulsive masturbation is a good example of an anxiety-reduction strategy. Parents can control food and alcohol, but it is difficult to stop a young person from masturbating. Other forms of physical and sexual abuse intensify poor self esteem and the need for relief from fear."

Treatment of depressive mood and anxiety related disorders

While counseling is essential, an early step to consider is medication. Medication to treat depressed mood and anxiety related disorders include multiple brands and types of Selective Serotonin Reuptake Inhibitors (SSRIs). They work to order the brain's transmission of serotonin from one synapse to the next. Many sexually addicted men initially reject the use of medication because they are fearful of the need to rely on the medication for the long-term or for life. Some fear they will become addicted to medication. While some may need long term medication therapy, most are able to "level the playing field" of their brain within six months to a year.

The phrase, "level the playing field," is meaningful and important. Depressed mood and anxiety-related disorders make it impossible for the man to see the world as hopeful. Depressed mood and anxiety foster negativity. When negativity is prominent in his life, he cannot see how he can change his behaviors. Medication is an important step for many sexually addicted men because it allows the brain to function normally and thus create a "level playing field" on top of which therapy can build a new reality.

Different medications are also available for anxiety-prone men. Again, depressed and anxiety-ridden men need mental stability to address behaviors, thinking, and relationships during their recovery journey.

Sexual thinking and fantasy

Sexually addicted men live in their heads. Processing sexually stimulating thinking and fantasy is part of their acting-out cycle. No true recovery is possible until the addict is willing to address and change what he allows his brain to process. Triggers for sexual thinking and fantasy are often images, real, or internet-based. However, the main sources of stimulation are images he keeps in the sexual file cabinet in his head from previous sexual encounters or material. It will take a lifetime of commitment to clean out the file cabinet in his head. Fortunately, as time goes by, nature helps to shed some of the material from the file cabinet. Ultimately, the man is well served to put a lock on the file cabinet.

Paradoxically, your partner may be encouraged to engage in sexual thinking and fantasy about you. Your partner does not feel guilt or remorse after engaging in loving marital relations. In most cases, sexual thinking and fantasy about you causes no harm. In fact, it may displace some of the illicit images he stores in his file cabinet. Part of sexual healing is to restore his relationship with you.

There is one caveat. Some men are sexually addicted to their wives and see them only as a solution to their lust. Bill read the Bible and took to heart his understanding of scripture. In his view, his wife was to be available when he needed her. Unfortunately, Bill's interpretation of the Bible was grossly out of proportion. He believed his wife should be compliant with sex in the morning, again when he got home from work, and many nights before sleep. Bill's wife tried to be a good wife but could not keep up with Bill's needs. She came to counseling in desperation. Bill refused to come. He said he did not have a problem.

The following questions may help you to determine if your partner is sexually addicted to you:

- Do you frequently feel as though your partner views you as an "object" for his pleasure?

- Do you find yourself consenting to sex to forestall his becoming angry or withdrawing?

- During sexual relations, is your partner's primary focus on his obtaining a satisfactory organism for himself? Do you often feel you are just along for the ride?

- Is his demand for sex so frequent that you feel used?

- Do you find that your partner is oblivious to relationship building and your sexual needs?

If you find you answered "yes" to many of these questions, individual and eventually marital counseling is in order for you and your husband. You need help to establish reasonable boundaries, and your husband needs help to address his sexual addiction, or at a minimum his sexual self-centeredness.

People can't live with change if there's not a changeless core inside them. The key to the ability to change is a changeless sense of who you are, what you are about and what you value.

Stephen Covey

Chapter Six

Codependency

To begin this chapter let me share a few thoughts with you.

- Clinical experience has shown that sexually-addicted men, when they marry, often marry into a codependent relationship. Codependency will affect the marriage and may affect his recovery. Both partners may find it beneficial to examine their role in the marriage.

- The term codependency was first coined in the Alcoholic Anonymous community. As it relates to sexual addiction, I define codependency as the propensity of marriage partners, where one of the partners is sexually addicted, to look for happiness or the lack of contentment based on the behavior of the partner. In simpler terms, each partner expects the other partner to cause their happiness. Melody Beattie (1992), a well known author in the field of codependency defines codependency as:

- "A codependent person is one who has let another person's behavior affect him or her, and who is obsessed with controlling that person's behavior."

- For the sexually addicted male, there is a clear road map to codependency. We noted earlier that the sexually addicted man did not have a nourishing relationship with his father—and in some cases, with his mother, when his mother assumed the characteristics of the paternal role in the family. Bradshaw (1988) relates:

- "Co-dependence is the most common family illness because it is what happens to anyone in any kind of the dysfunctional family. In every dysfunctional family, there is a primary stressor. This could be Dad's drinking or work addiction; Mom's hysterical control of everyone's feelings; Dad or Mom's physical or verbal violence; a family member's actual sickness or hypochondriasis; Dad or Mom's early death; their

56

divorce; Dad or Mom's moral/religious righteousness; Dad or Mom's sexual abuse. Anyone, who becomes controlling in the family to the point of being experienced as a threat by the other members, initiates the dysfunction."

- Again, the vast majority of sexually addicted men grew up in a dysfunctional family, often abusive, and most often with parents who were codependent themselves. It is natural for the sexually addicted man, when he seeks a partner, to find one who also experienced dysfunction and codependency in her family.

- Perhaps, as you read Bradshaw's description of codependency you will find elements of it that relate to you.

This chapter is not intended to assess blame on one or both partners. It merely conveys the reality that is found in many relationships involving a sexually addicted person. If after you read this chapter, you believe you are in a codependent relationship, then you are fortunate in your recognition. With knowledge comes power, and the choice to change what is not working in your relationship.

To explore how codependency affects marriages where the male is sexually addicted, we have two stories. The stories include many of the characteristics found in codependent relationships.

Jim and Barbara's story

Codependency characteristics are often evident before marriage.

Jim dated while he was in high school for social conformity. Since he had not witnessed respectful interactions between his parents, his relationship skills were also lacking. He did not know what it meant to get to know and appreciate a person of the opposite sex. Outside of school dances and similar functions, his social contact focused primarily on "making out." While "making out" never progressed beyond heavy petting, it was not for the lack of desire on his part.

Barbara also dated in high school. The man she dated was several years older and was in the military. For her, the relationship was safe because of the distance and infrequency of face to face contact. Having experienced a dysfunctional family environment, she too lacked understanding of a healthy relationship. She had a sense of loneliness because she often fought with her parents.

Jim and Barbara's parents were alike in many ways. Neither set of parents showed much affection. Jim's father was an alcoholic. Barbara and Jim felt their parents loved them, but external signs of affection were rare. When Jim left for college, the message he believed his parents sent was: anything short of a high level of performance was unacceptable. Barbara's motivation was more based on an internal perception that her parents would not love her if she did not succeed in her academic pursuits.

Barbara and Jim met at college. The college sponsored mixers for incoming freshman, and upperclassmen were invited to attend. Jim felt an immediate attraction to Barbara. To him, she had all the physical attributes that met his criteria for an attractive girl. He felt she was a bit naïve, but thought it was cute. On the other hand, while she thought Jim was reasonably attractive, she was not particularly interested in dating him. She had not planned to get involved with a college man because her studies were more important to her.

Jim invited Barbara to campus social affairs and fraternity parties. The first several times she turned him down. She finally agreed to go to a fraternity mixer. By this time, Jim was sexually attracted to Barbara. In fact, he had a number of erotic dreams that included Barbara. Jim began to plot ways to manipulate Barbara into a sexual relationship to satisfy his needs. Several months after their initial encounter, their relationship turned sexual. Once sexual activity entered into their relationship, neither seemed to put a priority on developing a strong non-sexual friendship. The glue that held the relationship together was physical and emotional dependency on each other.

Jim and Barbara dated for several years before they married. During this time, Jim's sexual needs continued to grow while Barbara tried to satisfy her need to be loved by giving into Jim's need.

Codependency characteristics flourish in marriage.

Jim and Barbara married and began a family. A year or so into the marriage, it became very apparent to Barbara that Jim was very self-centered and manipulative. His needs always seemed to come first. Joint decisions were often the product of Jim's persuasion. While he was a good economic provider, as a loving companion, he was far from ideal. Barbara felt very alone in the marriage and focused all her attention on raising their children. She tried numerous times to talk to him about her needs and her perception of a loving marriage. He repeatedly made promises to do better but did not do so. His perception was, as long as he provided a good economic subsistence for the family, he fulfilled his end of the bargain. Because he felt that Barbara constantly suggested ways in which he needed to improve, he shied away from give and take discussions because he feared he would see himself as a failure. Jim and Barbara grew apart in their marriage.

More than a decade into their marriage, Barbara learned that Jim had been unfaithful. Jim had marital affairs with several women at work and was addicted to pornography. In one long evening he confessed all of his transgressions and begged for Barbara's forgiveness. Jim insisted he would become a new man. Jim initially felt relieved that his greatest and most shameful secrets were exposed. The stress of leading a secret, dual life had become almost intolerable.

His promise to become a new man was short lived. He kept a secret stash of pornographic material for his periodic fix. In the deep recesses of his mind he reasoned he could, as he had done in the past, manipulate Barbara into accepting his promise to change his ways—and move on. Not this time! Barbara now recognized his manipulative behavior, and was not satisfied with his explanations, or his promises. Barbara was angry and decided she was not going to let Jim get away with what he had done to her and their family. She embarked on a plan to hold him accountable to his promise to change his behavior.

Jim wondered if the cure was not worse than the disease. He contemplated leaving Barbara but was terrified with the thought of being alone, and isolated from his children. He hoped that Barbara's fury would abate with time, but he was wrong.

Barbara also wondered whether she wanted to stay in the marriage. "Was it worth it," she asked herself? She contemplated leaving Jim, but was confounded by the thought of being financially insecure, and having to raise the children by herself. She convinced herself to stay until the children were in college. She made plans to get a job so she could grow financially independent. She saw Jim as a selfish "bastard" who was out to get his sexual needs met notwithstanding the total disregard for the marriage covenant. While she did not put it in terms of "punishment," she felt he had it coming when she monitored his every move. She had given up hope of ever trusting him again. And yet, deep down she felt she needed him, and the security that he provided. She saw Jim as a pathetic sex monger and herself as the victim of his total selfishness.

Jim and Barbara's marriage had hit rock bottom. Both were very angry people living under the same roof and incapable of seeing a way out of their dysfunctional relationship.

Epilog

Jim and Barbara were living in a codependent destructive world. Both were living under false premises. Jim thought his future happiness lay in Barbara agreeing to love him for whom he was without her trying to change him. Barbara saw her future happiness as a product of a reinvented Jim, and she was going to take charge of his reinvention.

Barbara was not going to be successful in changing Jim. Only Jim could change Jim. Sex could no longer be his greatest need. Jim's good friend suggested he consider getting help. On his own volition, Jim entered sex addiction counseling, and participated in an accompanying

Twelve-Step program. Jim's healing would take time, and he would have to grieve the damage he had done to himself, and to all those around him.

Marital therapy would be needed to reestablish trust, friendship, and a spiritual connection in the marriage. The healing journey will take years. Since Jim and Barbara contemplated divorce, if they don't invest fully in the program, they are doomed to repeat the same failures in any subsequent marriage. Ultimately, with therapy and commitment they can find the relationship both want and need in their present marriage.

Codependency characteristics in Jim and Barbara's marriage

The following are characteristics of codependency found in Jim and Barbara's story. You may or may not find yourselves in their story, but the principles set below mirror the experiences of many couples where the male is sexually addicted.

Characteristic # 1

The origin of codependency is found in a child's dysfunctional family.

Parents of codependent children are often codependent themselves, as were Jim and Barbara's parents. The traits are handed down, that is, taught to each succeeding generation. The parents of the codependent children are ill equipped to provide emotional nourishment to their children. Instead, dysfunctional families abound in addiction, narcissism, and the inability to show love to their children. When parents are internally focused on their own problems, they are ill equipped to build healthy relationships with their children. They can't give what they don't have.

Jim's father was an alcoholic. As such, he was not present to the developmental needs of his son. Jim learned from his father how to be self-centered. He learned that earning his father's love was based on his performance. His father looked to Jim to succeed where he perceived he failed in life. Jim's mother was a codependent enabler of her husband's alcoholism, that is, she continued to purchase alcohol for her husband. Jim could not get his emotional needs met from his family of origin. While he was unable to codify it as a child, as an adult he recognized that he was emotionally abandoned by his parents. His emotional deficiency led him to focus on satisfying his needs without regard to the needs of those around him.

From his parents, Jim also learned to manipulate others into meeting his needs. He used dominance to trump normal healthy interactions in his relationships. He was unable to be a friend and have empathy for others.

Jim was also sexually abused as a child at the hands of an older sibling. As he grew older, he turned to sexual stimulation for feelings of well being. He substituted sexual satisfaction for friendship and respect in his relationships.

Barbara's father was emotionally distant from his family. His work, and weekend golf, took precedence over his family. If he had a choice, he chose to be absent from his wife and children. When Barbara was a teenager, her mother often talked about wanting to leave her husband, but never did so. Barbara now recognizes that her parents were in a codependent relationship. Barbara did not experience a sense of well being from her parents. She felt she had to earn parental love. Among her siblings, she was the caretaker and the responsible child.

Both Jim and Barbara were predestined to enter into a codependent relationship.

Characteristic # 2

Children of codependent dysfunctional families have ill-formed or incomplete personalities.

Adult behavior, either intentionally or not, builds on the dysfunctional personality traits learned in the family of origin.

Jim often felt deficient in his social skills, and questioned his self-worth. Because of his low self-esteem, he often wondered if anyone really could love him. Nevertheless, his distorted thinking led him to equate sex with a feeling of being loved. Through his previous experience with sexual stimulation, he sought mood escalation by repeated attempts to manipulate his high school and college girl friends. It never occurred to Jim that there was much more to a relationship than making out. After all, he reasoned, if a girl would participate in sexual activity with him, surely they loved each other.

Barbara's hole in the soul was her need to be loved. In response to the attention she received from Jim, she allowed herself to be manipulated into an early sexual relationship. From time to time, she felt sex occupied far too much of their relationship. Several times she attempted to establish what she considered more healthy boundaries. She was no match for Jim's manipulative skills.

Jim's attraction to Barbara focused on her attractive body parts. He lacked the insight needed to focus on her personality, and her personhood. He felt that the essence of a steady relationship was to have Barbara depend on him. While Barbara frequently felt uneasy, she also lacked the skills to objectively evaluate their relationship. She bought into depending on him for an active college environment. After all, he was a fraternity brother, and she wore his pin.

Characteristic # 3

In marriage, codependency fosters pain and negativity.

Once married, Jim's eyes began to wander. He needed the thrill of pursuing a new conquest. He began to repeat the cycle he began with Barbara while they were in college. Jim lacked marriage skills, and his pursuits outside of the marriage bed further distanced him from providing the emotional nourishment Barbara so dearly needed.

Barbara substituted her desire for marital happiness by focusing her attention on her children. Her friends saw her as an outstanding and dedicated mother. She tried to meet her children's every need. Barbara transferred her dependence on Jim to dependence on her children for her emotional well being. She tried to fill the hole in her soul by forming a loving relationship with her children. However, children are unable to return love as would a healthy adult.

Jim continued to insist on sex with Barbara, who was fearful of saying no because she feared Jim's anger. Barbara felt disconnected from Jim. She gave him what he wanted, but she felt she was simply paying dues.

Characteristic # 4

Fear, shame, anger, and depressed mood are all companions of codependency.

Jim continued to live in two worlds—one foot in his sexual fantasy world and one foot inside the home. While he believed he was clever enough to not get caught, he realized that his life was out of control, and getting worse. He was ashamed, and lived in a low-grade depressed mood. He knew that his relationship with Barbara had gone from good to bad but had no idea how to change it. He had no intention of giving up his best friend, sex. After all, as many sexually addictive men reason, a man needs some pleasure in life.

When Barbara learned of Jim's close held secrets, she felt conflicting emotions. On the one hand, she was relieved that her suspicions were real, and she was not crazy. On the other hand, she was outraged, and felt great anger. She was also dominated by fear. She was fearful she would be left totally alone in life: what would become of her and the children? How could anyone understand the intense feeling of betrayal she felt? She was so depressed that getting out of bed each day, eating, and caring for the children seemed like monumental tasks.

Characteristic # 5

Codependency is part of the problem.

For Jim and Barbara, codependency was an integral part of their marriage. Jim depended on his ability to manipulate Barbara so he could continue to get his needs met. Barbara depended on her anger to respond to Jim's betrayal of their marriage contract.

Neither would be successful.

Both would benefit from counseling. Jim needed to address his addictive behavior. Barbara would have done well to seek counseling to heal the consequences of her marital relationship. They both needed help to deal with the present crisis, and to help support the family.

Joe and Alice's story

Joe, a mid-level executive, had multiple affairs during his twenty years of marriage to Alice. It was usual for Joe to have more than one affair going at the same time. While his marriage to Alice provided him with two wonderful children, he continued his liaisons. He said, "I don't feel particularly close to Alice. She does her thing, and I do mine."

Joe protected his computer and e-mail account with passwords. One evening he inadvertently left his e-mail account open. Alice stumbled onto Joe's e-mail exchanges with his ladies. Pandemonium ensued.

Alice went to Joe and demanded full disclosure. Joe complied, but refused to give sufficient details to satisfy Alice. Joe felt he did not want to cause more pain than he had already caused. He also talked about the shame of his behavior, and his fear that Alice would leave him if she knew the details. Alice wanted a full accounting of all his transgressions, and she wanted him to keep her abreast of his behavior and thinking on a daily basis. She was angry and terrified. She felt betrayed, and was concerned about the future of their marriage, and the raising of their children.

Neither Joe nor Alice wanted a divorce but the bond between them had been fractured. Joe said that for years, he wanted to let Alice in on his most guarded secrets of infidelity, but feared she would try to fix him, or leave him. In fact, his fears became a reality. Alice, in her despondency, did everything she could think of to hold Joe accountable to her perception of a good marriage. In her zeal to monitor Joe, she obtained his credit card and telephone records for as many years as she could. On a continuing basis, she questioned any call that was not readily recognizable. She constantly accused him of going back to being unfaithful. She insisted on obtaining the phone number for each of the women with whom he had been unfaithful. She called every one of them to make it clear that Joe was no longer available. She embarrassed him by talking about what a rotten person he was to anyone who would listen—at his work, church, and community.

Alice continued to demand more information, and frequently asked questions about one or more of his affairs. Periodically Joe would provide the detail of an affair, which then resulted in Alice's berating him for the content of the detail. After each disclosure, she yelled that she could not trust him, because she did not know how much more he had not told her.

They discussed their behavior in a joint marital therapy session. Alice and Joe made promises to change, but they did not. Their marriage therapist speculated that Alice had a hole in her soul related to sexual abuse as a child. In other words, she had her own shame. Shame binds Joe to Alice. Unless they deal with the roots of their dysfunction from childhood, it is unlikely the marriage will survive.

The other side of the coin.

Perhaps you identify with the steps Alice took to reclaim her partner. After all, what was wrong with her taking positive action? Why shouldn't she demand accountability from him? Why shouldn't she demand that he confess his transgressions in real time, so she could know how sincere he was in his promise to change? After all, she is the victim of his profound selfishness—putting his needs ahead of everything dear and sacred to the marriage contract.

The answer?

Alice is justified in her anger. However, if Joe is not committed to hold himself accountable to changing his behavior, Alice's efforts are headed for frustration and divorce. It is Joe who has to see that putting his sexual needs ahead of all else has a dim future.

Alice's actions add to Joe's shame. Sexual addiction is a shame-based disease. While hardly an excuse to justify acting-out behavior, shame, and feelings of worthlessness, often contribute to acting out. Sexually addicted men self medicate negative feelings. One of the tasks sexually addicted men address during recovery is exposing their sense of shame to the light of day. Group and Twelve Step programs seek to counter negativity which exists in their lives. An essential step is to learn to live at the forty-point benchmark level by taking positive steps to come out of isolation, allowing shame to recede, and to forgo living in low-grade depression. Perhaps one could argue that Joe deserves to feel guilt and shame, but doing so will not help him on his recovery journey.

Visual picture of Joe and Alice's codependency relationship

Picture two elevators side by side: Joe occupies one and Alice the other. When Alice's elevator is on the tenth floor, Joe's elevator is in the basement. When Joe's elevator is in the basement, he sees himself as the errant child and he looks up to Alice on the tenth floor and sees a scornful mother. Joe gives Alice the power to chastise, for he believes he deserves it, but he intensely resents her for doing so. Alice takes the power given to her and dutifully scolds and punishes. She is no longer the spouse, but has taken the role of Jim's dysfunctional mother.

They ride their elevators to the opposite levels. Alice's elevator is now in the basement and Joe's is on the tenth floor. Alice sees herself as the victim of Joe's self-centeredness. She sees his behavior as willful, destructive to the marriage, and selfish. She sees him in a superior position—doing his own thing without regard to the consequences, particularly to the marriage. Joe supports her vision by continuing to put his sexual needs first.

Joe and Alice continue to ride their respective elevators, alternating between the basement and tenth floor. As they ride, they get more and more angry, and blame each other for their predicament.

What needs to change?

In simplistic terms, both Joe and Alice would do well to ride their elevators to the fifth floor, get off, and face one another.

Ideally, Joe admits he is powerless to stop his behavior—it has become unmanageable.

Alice rejects the role of Joe's mother. Alice tells Joe, "It is not my job to change you. That is your challenge." If so inclined, she can tell him, "I will pray for you. If you would like a friendly ear while you are in therapy, I may agree to listen, but I am not willing to try to be your accountability partner or make suggestions."

Alice may choose to deal with the origins of her codependent behavior in individual or group therapy.

Joe's fifth floor position is to thank Alice and to commit to counseling. His therapist will likely also recommend he attend one or multiple Twelve-Step programs on a regular basis.

You and codependency addressed

In a healthy marriage, partners see themselves neither in a superior position nor as the victim, but as equals. Each takes individual responsibility to grow in wisdom. The male's goal is to accept that he has a problem which he commits to address. The woman's goal is to accept that she, too, has issues that she could address. They support each other in a quest to become whole, and shun the paralyzing effects of shame.

In a codependent relationship, each partner's identity lies outside of the self. Each depends on the other to provide wholeness. Neither is independent in the relationship. For example, if you would like to change your partner's behavior, you are saying, "For me, happiness lies in how my partner can change, not on how I function independently." In a codependent relationship, both parties want to be in charge but neither party feels that they are, and yet, each party feels the other is in charge.

A practical way to change your codependent response is: instead of giving advice, ask your partner how he is dealing with such and such a situation. Thank him for his thoughts and tell him you will pray for him. Tell him you have issues you want to work on as well. Tell him you are open to hear what he has learned and interested in what he wants to share. Don't let yourself engage in a codependent response.

If your partner attempts to give you advice, ask him to tell you how it would change him if you followed his advice. Thank him for sharing, and tell him that you need to pray on what you heard. You are now free to either make the change or not. Just because someone else wants something doesn't mean they are going to get it.

The difference in the above behavior is: you have introduced loving independence.

Two more considerations

- While it is far from ideal, clinical experience has shown that the majority of men who enter sexual addiction therapy do so because their spouse has set a boundary that includes getting help.

- The vast majority of men cannot follow the recovery road by themselves. For the most part, any reasoning which purports to the opposite is a rationalization, and contains elements of manipulation.

What else can I read about codependency?

The following books are well worth reading.

Codependent No More: How to Stop Controlling Others and Start Caring for Yourself by Melody Beattie

Hazelden Publishing; 2nd edition (September 1, 1992)

From the book cover:

> "By its nature, alcoholism and other compulsive disorders create victims out of everyone close to the afflicted person. Whether the person you love is an alcoholic, a gambler, a foodaholic, a workaholic, a sexaholic, a criminal, a rebellious teenager, or a neurotic parent, this book is for you—the codependent. This inspiring overview of codependency by Melody Beattie, a recovering alcoholic and former chemical dependency counselor, details its characteristics, where the behavior comes from, and how it affects us and those around us. Offering hope and guidance, *Codependent No More* discusses several options to controlling behavior and helps us understand that letting go will set us free."

Facing Codependence: What It Is, Where It Comes from, How It Sabotages Our Lives by Pia Melody with Andrea Wells Miller and J. Keith Miller.

Harper & Row; 1 edition (May 17, 1989)

From the book cover:

> "In this fresh new look at Codependence, Pia Melody traces the origins of this illness back to childhood, describing a whole range of emotional, spiritual, intellectual, physical, and sexual abuses. Because of these earlier experiences, codependent adults lack the skills necessary to lead mature lives and have satisfying relationships."

Bradshaw On: The Family: A New Way of Creating Solid Self-Esteem by John Bradshaw

HCI; Revised edition (April 1, 1990)

From the book cover:

> ". . . John Bradshaw focuses on the dynamics of the family, how the rules and attitudes learned while growing up becoming encoded with each family member. As 96% of all families are to some degree emotionally impaired, the unhealthy rules we are now living by are handed down from one generation to another and ultimately to society at large. Our society is sick because our families are sick. And our families are sick because we are living by inherited roles that we never wrote."

Women, Sex, and Addiction: A Search for Love and Power by Charlotte Sophia Kasl

Harper Paperbacks; 1st, First Edition (July 5, 1990)

From the book cover:

> "In our society, sex can easily become the price men and women pay for love and the illusion of security. A woman who seeks a sense of personal power and an escape from the pain may use sex and romance as a way to feel in control, just as alcoholics use alcohol; but sex never satisfies her longing for love and self worth. In this wise and compassionate book, Charlotte Sophia Kasl, shows women how they can learn to experience their sexuality as a source of love and positive power and sex as an expression that honors the soul as well as the body."

The internet will provide more descriptive reviews of these books as well as multiple sources for purchasing.

Sexually Addicted men often live in a fantasy world. For the most part, they believe in the illogical: I will never get caught and if I am caught, I will minimize my sexual behavior. The following cartoon by Zuzu Galifianakis (2011) gives us insight into male thinking. The logic expressed in the cartoon is never so on target than when it applies to pornography addiction, the subject of the next chapter.

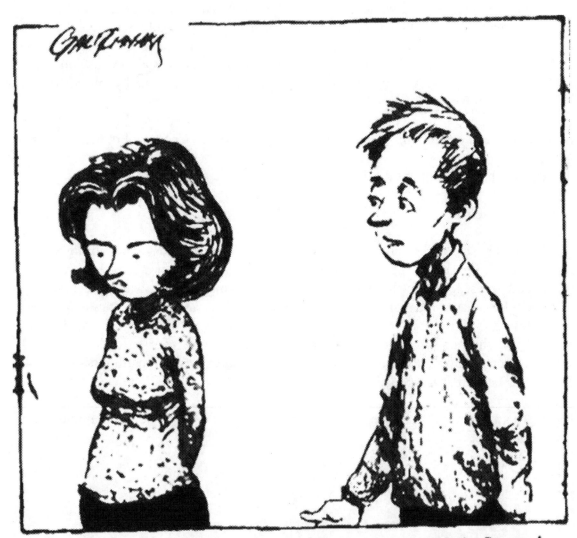

Self-respect is the root of discipline; the sense of dignity grows with the ability to say no to oneself.

Abraham J. Heschel

Treat your mind like a bad neighborhood—don't go there alone.

Source Unknown

Chapter Seven

Pornography

Pornography is the millstone around the neck of a sexually addicted man. Perhaps the number one reason sexually-addicted men enter therapy is to deal with addiction to pornography. Most have been caught viewing pornography online by their wife, significant other, or employer.

Men crave returning to the secrecy of sexual stimulation that occurred during childhood. They mistakenly believe they can go online and enjoy their own secret world of sexual stimulation and never get caught. A pattern repeated by many men is to stay up late—after their wives have gone to sleep—and search the internet for sexually stimulating images.

Bart's story

Bart believed viewing online pornography did not affect his marriage. Bart was an upwardly mobile young executive and often took work home. He had an agreement with his wife that he would not do office work while she and the children were awake. After Bart's wife retired for the evening, Bart went online. He would spend an hour or two attending to office work, but then succumbed to the temptation to view pornographic material. He felt he deserved to reward himself, for he was an outstanding breadwinner and his wife did not seem to need sexual activity as much as he did. He looked forward to viewing pornography and subsequent masturbation.

His wife was a sound sleeper and never disturbed his late night sessions on the computer. That was, until one night when she walked in on him, and saw what she called "sick" images on his computer. Not only did she see the images on his computer, but he was in the process of masturbating when she walked in.

Bart's wife, like any normal wife, was traumatized by her husband's behavior. She told him that unless he got help, their relationship was likely over. Now Bart was devastated. Bart entered therapy, but found the road back to sexual sobriety more difficult than he expected. After a year of therapy, Bart continued three times a week attendance at a Twelve Step program to keep himself straight. He also found that an exercise program helped him maintain a better mental disposition. Having been discovered, Bart said, was initially the worst thing that could have happened to him. He now realizes it was the opportunity for life changing choices, and a far better relationship with his wife.

Men also go online from their computers at work and believe they will not get caught.

Bill's story

Bill was an IT guy who believed he could defeat any filter or tracking tools used by his employer. His employer was a State government. However, it was not the controls that his employer put on the system that caused Bill to lose his "dream" position. One Friday afternoon he was called into his supervisor's office and told to pack up his things. He was no longer an employee. His supervisor explained to him that a female coworker filed a sexual harassment complaint after she observed pornographic images on Bill's computer as she passed by his work cubicle. Bill was devastated. His wife was outraged. The family was in crisis. A major problem faced by the family was paying for the medical care of their disabled son. Bill was able to obtain freelance work to barely keep the family afloat. Bill, and his family, paid a high price for the lure of pornographic images.

Art's story

Art's employer made it clear, anyone caught viewing pornography at the work site would be fired. Art was a highly specialized engineer, and thought, no matter what he did, he would never be fired. His company needed his expertise. Art's pattern of behavior was to view online pornography after his coworkers left for the day. He got caught, and was told by his boss that he had one more chance. He failed to take stock of the warning. He was subsequently fired for his activity on a company computer. Art entered therapy to try to convince his boss he was serious about changing his behavior. Art learned it was not his boss whom he needed to satisfy, but himself. He made good progress in therapy and is employed by another company.

Definition of pornography

Defining pornography for universal acceptance is nearly impossible. You may wish to go online to find a definition that meets your standards. For the purposes of this book we use an over-simplified definition.

> Pornography is any sexually stimulating material or language that is used by a sexually addicted person to foster sexual stimulation.

We understand that sexually stimulating material may be used by married couples. Nevertheless, even such use falls within our definition if the focus of the sexually addicted man is more on the stimulating images than on his wife. Some find it hard to believe that pornography of any type is healthy within the marriage. Why does a man or a woman need external materials to facilitate sexual arousal? In such cases, other issues are at work which precludes marital intimacy. They need to be addressed.

The simplistic approach toward a definition means any material a man uses to foster sexual stimulation is pornography for him. As indicated earlier, pornography may or may not be the type found at an adult bookstore. One man found lingerie ads in newspapers and catalogs to be his form of pornography. Another man found images of large-breasted women to be tantalizing, and he never went further than his everyday TV shows. Bill found women with long slender necks stimulating. His subway ride back and forth to work was his pornography studio. In the final analysis, pornography is what each man finds stimulating. What stimulates one man may not stimulate another man and vice versa.

While more classifications of pornography exist, pornography is usually found in the following mediums: literature, photos, internet, sculptures, drawings, paintings, animation, sound recordings, movies, TV, films, DVDs, Blu-ray, pay-for-view, videos, or video games. Let us look at a few of these.

> **Literature and photos:** The spicy novel with sexually stimulating stories and scenes has been around for ages. In the past century, men's magazines such as *Playboy* and *Penthouse* became popular and the source of initiation into the world of sex for many boys. While these magazines do not violate the Supreme Court's standard of obscenity, adult bookstores sell even more sexually explicit magazines that comes close to violating the Supreme Court standard of obscenity.

> **Film, DVD, and video:** From the midpoint of the previous century, pornography came off the printed page into movement and even more explicit sexual enactment. Adult bookstores thrived on making available first 8mm movies followed by videocassettes and then DVDs and Blu-rays. Material sold by adult book stores generally contains hard-core pornography and illicit acts. Adult bookstores look forward to visiting conventioneers who find a trip away from home as an opportunistic time to purchase future pleasure.

TV and pay-for-view: In recent years, the man who subscribes to a full range of cable or satellite TV channels has available more pornography than he could ever digest. The only difficulty he has is finding a time to view his material so he does not get caught. One man said he set his alarm clock for a predawn hour so he could watch sexually stimulating material before going to work. Men who travel frequently may find pay-for-view movies in their hotel room are their downfall.

Movies: It's difficult to go to a movie theater these days without being exposed to sexually explicit scenes and nudity. While they are acceptable in today's society, they can cause a man to retain images in his head and to mentally process them later, along with masturbation.

Immodest dress: Both women and men dress for attention. Clothing and how it is worn can be alluring or sexually revealing. Young people may or may not recognize that the way they dress will cause sexual arousal—very toxic to a sexually addicted man. One man remarked, "I need blinders when I drive across a college campus. Some young women wear less clothing than allowed in a doctor's exam room."

Internet: The internet is the ultimate presentation of pornography in today's society. While many web sites entice men to pay for more explicit images, plenty of material is available for free. More disturbing is available material that exploits children. If depression was the mental health common cold of the last century, internet pornography is the pneumonia of this century. Of greater concern is the number of young people and teenagers who have unfettered access to sexually stimulating material on the internet.

Cybersex: Cybersex has as its common elements the use of a computer, internet access, expected anonymity, and sexually provocative material to generate arousal followed most often by masturbation. Multiple venues exist such as dial-a-porn, e-mail, chat rooms, live video streams, instant messaging, postings to social networks (like Facebook), visual images of real or graphically generated persons, and interactive sex through a web cam.

Statistics on pornography

Pornography is huge and it is growing. Unfortunately, more children are being exposed to pornography and thus are potential for addiction. The following tables give insight into just how insidious just one form of sexual stimulation has become—internet pornography.

United States Pornography Revenues
Revenue from pornography is more than $97 billion a year. The pornography industry has larger revenues than the revenues of the top technology companies **combined:** Microsoft, Google, Amazon, eBay, Yahoo, Apple, Netflix, and Earthlink. Revenue from pornography in the United States exceeds the combined revenues of ABC, CBS, and NBC

Pornography Time Statistics
Every second—$3,075.64 is being spent on pornography
Every second—28,258 internet users are viewing pornography
Every 39 minutes: a new pornographic video is being created in the United States

Internet Pornography Statistics	
Pornographic web sites	4.2 million (12% of total web sites)
Pornographic pages	**420 million**
Daily pornographic search engine requests	68 million (25% of search engine requests)
Daily Gnutella "child pornography" requests	116,000
Web sites offering illegal child pornography	**100,000**
Youths who received sexual solicitation	1 in 7

Children Internet Pornography Statistics	
Average age of first internet exposure to pornography	**11 years-of-age**
15-17 year olds having multiple hard-core exposures	80%
8-16 year olds having viewed porn online	**90% (most while doing homework)**

Adult Internet Pornography Statistics	
Percentage of internet users who view pornography	42.7%
Men admitting to accessing pornography at work	20%
US adults who regularly visit internet pornography web sites	40 million
Promise Keeper men who viewed pornography in the last week	**53%**
Christians who said pornography is a major problem in the home	**47%**

(Family Safe Media, 2012)

The problem that pornography is causing in our society is staggering and growing. Just think: if while you were at church this past Sunday, you looked left and right, one of the two people you greeted could have said pornography is a problem in their home. If 53% of Promise Keeper men admit to viewing pornography last week, your partner is far from alone.

Internet pornography content

When one thinks of a man viewing pornography on the internet, it is reasonable to think of him viewing women in some form of normal sexuality. The reality is the internet provides both normal sexuality as well as a large menu of perverted sexuality. Briefly, examples of perverted sexual behavior are bestiality, sadomasochism (S & M), sexual violence including sadomasochism and rape, exploitation of children, and other perversions that go beyond the need to describe them here.

A therapist asked the men in his sexual addiction therapy group to disclose the nature of the material they viewed on line. The purpose of asking them to disclose internet pornography images of choice was to explore a connection between current interests and a disturbing event that occurred during childhood. When such a connection is identified, it may be possible to reduce the addictive power of the current interest.

Glenn's story

Glenn was a city boy who was sent to his uncle's farm one summer when he was about the age of ten. To the farm boy, animal copulation is part of everyday business. His cousin realized that Glenn had never seen animals mate. He took Glenn to the pasture one day when the veterinarian was on hand to breed a stallion with a prized mare. Glenn was not ready for what he witnessed. He was sexually stimulated and confused by seeing the mating process. He remembers dreaming about what he saw a number of times over the next several years. In fact, he became fascinated with human copulation as well.

Glenn, as an adult, stumbled on an internet site that featured bestiality. He returned to that site and others like it for several years. He never understood why this perverted act stimulated him. While in therapy he was able to see the connection between what happened at age ten and what kept him fixated as an adult.

If your partner is addicted to internet pornography, some steps are available to help him, and perhaps other members of your family. For the man who is not computer savvy, a number of commercial software programs are available to block access to pornography. Type in "blocking software" into your internet browser search bar and you'll find multiple alternatives.

For the man who is computer savvy enough to get around internet blocking programs, software entitled *Covenant Eyes* is excellent. This software goes beyond blocking access to web sites the user wishes to access. It provides a weekly report to a person designated by the user to receive the report. The report details every site the user accessed during the week of reference. (Covenant Eyes, 2012) can be found on http: //www.covenanteyes.com/

Live the life you've dreamed

David Henry Thoreau

Chapter Eight

The Recovery Journey

The books, *In Search of Recovery: A Christian Man's Guide*, Becker (2010) and, *In Search of Recovery Workbook: A Christian Man's Guide*, Becker (2010) provide detailed information for the man who wishes to overcome sexual addiction. An outline of the information found in the guides is presented here to give you an overview of issues your partner may wish to address in therapy. The books are available from: http://gentlepath.com/ and from sexaddiction.sexaddictionhelpbooks.com

Acknowledging the problem

Recovery begins with acknowledging the problem. For many men, acknowledging the problem is not as simple as it sounds. Frequently, men enter therapy in order to placate a wife or significant other's outrage of having discovered their man's sexual behaviors outside the relationship. Agreeing to go to therapy may not be a commitment to change behavior. Denial of the seriousness of the problem, and thus the need for a solution is common. Usually, if the man stays with therapy, he overcomes denial and begins a true healing process.

It is not your job as the wife or significant other to convince the man of his need for commitment. His commitment will occur best during therapy and attending frequent Twelve Step sessions.

Hearing other men's stories in group therapy leads to awareness. He will hear he is neither alone in his addiction, nor as evil as he fears.

Awareness leads to choices

A therapist who works with sexually addicted men can almost see the light bulb go on. When the man begins to fully understand his behavior is causing problems to himself and his family, enlightenment has begun.

Ultimately, the man will face choices to change his lifestyle and ultimately his aberrant sexual behavior. Interestingly, long-term sexual healing is not just a matter of ending behavior; it is a matter of changing both the man's internal and external environment so the behavioral breeding ground is decimated.

An example of an internal environmental change is ending sexual thinking and fantasy. Sexual sobriety cannot be maintained unless the brain is taught to end tantalizing triggers.

An example of an external environmental change is addressing his chronically depressed mood. This is not simply saying, "I am a happy person." It means initiating and maintaining positive behaviors that foster a new outlook on life. It means choosing activities that foster living at the forty-point benchmark level. When a man chooses to live at the forty-point benchmark level, as discussed in chapter 5, he seeks uplifting scenarios such as daily exercise, frequent dates with his partner, a supportive male friend, and engages in other activities that improve relationships with his immediate, and extended family. Living at the forty-point benchmark level reduces chronic depressed mood, and lowers the propensity to act out sexually.

These examples are but some of the new steps your partner will want to pursue if he is committed to changing the addiction dance.

Commitment

In humor, a smoker might say, "I am committed to stop every time I put a cigarette out. I've done it thousands of times." For the sexually addicted man, the same phrase is not humorous. He has committed to himself to quit many times. The reason why the man is unable to maintain his commitment is because his internal and external environments have not changed. Internally he has not freed himself from sexual thinking and fantasy. Externally he has not freed himself from isolation and low-grade depression.

The man continues to struggle with temptations because he allows temptation to bounce around in his brain. The man continues to "white knuckle" his addiction. Temptation comes, the man struggles to rid himself of temptation, and then the man succumbs to temptation, over and over again. As long as he continues to "white knuckle" his recovery, his success will be problematical.

An alternative to "white knuckling" is called making a "high level commitment." The difference between "white knuckling" and "high level commitment" is a man's approach to the decision. In a "white knuckling" approach, the man does not eliminate the possibility of succumbing to temptation. As an example, when a man who likes to view pornography tells himself he will no longer look at pornographic magazines but does not destroy his collection, he is "white knuckling" his commitment. Hidden away are several choice magazines against the day he really needs a fix. Unfortunately, that day is not far away. In the example, if the man eliminated his whole collection and other stimulating sources of pornography (pornographic movies, CDs, and provocative cable channels, etc.) he rejects the source of temptation. A man who makes a "high level commitment" totally rejects the possibility of acting out.

It is not easy to explain to a sexually addicted man what a "high level commitment" looks like as contrasted to "white knuckling." Understanding comes with experience. He understands after he irrevocably commits himself to rejecting acting-out behavior. Once he experiences a "high level commitment," the impact of temptation changes. When a man "white knuckles' his recovery, he continually struggles to reject temptation, but often fails. When a man lives his "high level commitment," the struggle ends. Since he is totally committed to rejecting acting-out, and even thinking about it, temptation is immediately dismissed at its inception.

Recognition that addiction causes more pain than pleasure

Sexual stimulation leads to orgasm. The "high" of preparing for orgasm and the "rush" experienced during orgasm is as God intended, pleasurable. While a man will actually work to lengthen the experience, acting out is a relatively short time of intense feeling. Sooner or later, a recovering addict realizes time spent in pleasure as contrasted to time spent in shame and guilt is out of balance.

A man ultimately realizes it is impossible to be intimate with self and intimate in the marriage with the same intensity. Unfortunately, the addict reports intimacy with self is powerful because he is in control of the entire scenario. He needs no one's cooperation but himself. The most powerful sex organ is his brain. In therapy he begins to understand that, despite the pleasure of self-stimulation, his behavior is selfish, and often child-like. He begins to understand that his behavior ultimately causes pain to self and others.

You may ask, "How can sex be pleasurable and at the same time cause pain to a man? He obviously likes the feeling he experiences during orgasm. Where does the pain come in, and if there is pain, why didn't he stop long ago?"

Yes, he likes the euphoric feeling associated with orgasm and he repeats his acting-out behavior to duplicate the feeling. However, for many men the euphoric feeling is followed by feelings of guilt and shame. Such feelings remain until he begins his acting-out cycle again. (See Appendix B for a discussion of the acting-out cycle.) For the man for whom acting out has become a compulsive habit, the negative side of the acting-out cycle has become a "normal" consequence with which he lives. Since he hasn't experienced the joy of long-term sobriety, he lacks understanding. A sexually addicted man simply does not know what the alternative to acting out looks like. Acting out is the only sexual life he knows.

A competent therapist can help the man see that, in the long run, he experiences more pain than pleasure. A man in therapy said, "Why am I doing this to myself?"

Men who have spent many years in prison actually fear getting out because they don't know if they can adjust. Well, your partner has spent many years in the prison of sexual addiction. He, too, does not know what it will be like to live on the other side of addiction. An often heard comment from men in therapy is, "I don't know what it's like not to be sexually addicted. I don't know what normal looks like."

When a man in therapy begins to talk about how much pain his addiction is causing, relative to the short periods of pleasure he experiences during acting out, another light bulb goes on. His enlightenment is a significant milestone in his recovery.

During therapy, your partner should gain insight and experience a series of "light bulb" moments. Each one will bring him closer to long term sexual sobriety. If you are committed to listen to him during his therapy, you, too, can share in his insights and the joy of recovery. It is critical to his recovery and the health of your relationship that you care.

Addressing environmental temptation

We have noted several times that a critical step in recovery is to eliminate sexual thinking and fantasy. Other sources of sexual stimulation also need to be addressed. Without going into detail, a sexually addicted man will have to address: (That which needs to be addressed will differ from one man to another.)

- Putting blocking software on his computer. Many men learn to defeat blocking software. Covenant Eyes software provides an accountability report that provides information on every computer site visited. The way to beat the software is to stay away from offensive sites.

- Eliminating pay-for-view sexually stimulating channels.

- Learning to "bounce one's eyes" (The term "bouncing eyes" was popularized by Arterburn to mean a man needs to look away when he encounters a sexually stimulating image or person.) (Arterburn, 2000)

- Learning to change the channel when a provocative show or scene comes on.

- Saying "no" to pornography found in men's magazines, DVDs and Blu-ray videos, ads in newspapers, internet, etc.

- Saying "no" to participation in chat rooms, phone sex, massage parlors, strip joints, lap dancing, etc.

- Getting rid of "stash." (Stash is a man's stimulating material which is kept in secret for the day when he believes he needs to be rewarded with self-sex).

- Learning to focus on a woman's face rather than her "body parts."

- Understanding each woman (even a porn star) is somebody's mother, sister, daughter, or spouse.

These are but some examples men find they need to address. Each man has his own sexually stimulating triggers. Part of the recovery journey requires a man to make a rigorous inventory of that which begins his acting-out ritual.

A man may identify something he finds sexually stimulating that the world would not consider as sexual. For example, one man in therapy disclosed he found pictures of sailboats with cabins sexually stimulating but he had no idea why. He learned that the connection between a sexually stimulating image of a sailboat came from the sexual abuse he experienced on a sailboat as a child. Each time he saw a sailboat his internal child responded to the sense of arousal he experienced during his abuse. For him, once he understood the connection, it lessened the power of the stimulus. However, he found it was also helpful to stay away from pictures of sailboats with cabins, at least early in his recovery journey.

Choosing a healthy lifestyle

In chapter 5 we explored the link between a chronically depressed mood and acting out. In order to reduce the power of the disparity of living at the twenty-point benchmark and acting out at the fifty-point benchmark, the man must make conscious decisions to incorporate more forty-point benchmark activities into his life. Some of the activities men find helpful include:

- A weekly exercise program sufficient enough to achieve an "endorphin high." While an "endorphin high" is not as powerful as the high associated with orgasm, it does have legitimate substitute value.

- Incorporating healthy activities into one's life such as hiking, biking, softball, tennis, golf, soccer, etc. (Ideally some of these new healthy activities will be family or couple activities.)

- Plan ahead each week to participate in mood lifting activities with spouse, and or family.

- Develop a healthy relationship with a higher power or God. Sexually addicted men see God as distant in their life. Their God is often judgmental and rarely loving. Most sexually addicted men did not have a nourishing relationship with their biological father, thus they form an image of God that has the same characteristics as did their earthly father. His relationship with God is experienced as a mirror image of the one he had with his biological father. It is an extraordinary blessing for the man to realize God is his greatest cheerleader. God blesses his struggle; He does not condemn his failures.

- Volunteer to help others. A spiritual connection is often found in serving others. When the focus is switched from self to others, the vision of the world in which the man lives changes. Sexually addicted men are takers. Long term healing occurs when they become givers.

- Any new and positive behavior a man chooses to raise his mood in a healthy way.

Coming out of isolation

The sexually addicted man lives in a world where his focus is always internal. His most important need, and thus behavior, makes him feel euphoric for short periods of time. However, subsequent to acting out he returns to his twenty-point benchmark, his low-grade depressive mood, and thus isolation. Isolation is often a consequence of low-grade depression.

Some of the activities men find helpful to address isolation include:

Cultivate a strong male relationship. Because sexually addicted men live in shame, they find it impossible to let anyone get close to their secrets. Healthy, intimate relationships with other males are not part of the addicted man's world. One of the man's most difficult recovery tasks is to purposely cultivate a healthy relationship with another male. Such a relationship can serve to help break the shame-based isolation that characterizes the life of the man. The ultimate goal is to trust another male so he can confide his temptations and secrets. A place to look for a healthy male relationship, a male who can ultimately serve as an accountability partner, is in a Twelve Step program, church group, and/or a therapy group.

Improve relationships with family of origin. Since sexually addicted men are the product of dysfunctional families, relationships between parents and siblings are often damaged. Such damage leads to isolation. The addicted man believes he is alone in his dysfunction. When he begins to understand that his siblings, as well as his parents, carry the wounds of generational pain, he can gain empathy, and foster bonds with them. Men are encouraged to approach parents and siblings with the question, "What was it like for you to grow up in our/your family of origin?" This question is a good icebreaker and nonthreatening. Although it may take time, opening a dialogue with siblings and parents can be very therapeutic and heals destructive bonds.

Improve relationships with a spouse and children. Often a man feels a greater degree of intimacy outside the marriage than he experiences with a spouse and children. For the addicted man, intimacy equals sex. He has no concept of nonsexual intimacy. In fact, it is quite common to learn that in the relationship between a sexually addicted man and his future spouse, sexual activity entered the relationship early. Once sexual activity entered the relationship, the process of building friendship ended. The focus was on obtaining more sexual gratification, often by both partners. One of the reasons for suggesting a temporary hiatus in sexual relations is to allow time to go back and fill in the missing ingredients found in a healthy marital relationship. That means spending time talking, sharing nonsexual activities, sharing meals together, a weekly date, and just about any other activity which builds friendship in the marriage. Most men report a thrill when their partner becomes their best friend. When both partners in a marriage are able to say "yes" to many of the non-sexual intimacy statements below, isolation in the marriage will dissipate.

I know that I have intimacy in my marriage when:

- I consider my partner to be a very good listener.

- My partner understands how I feel.

- We have a good balance of leisure time spent together and separately.

- I look forward to spending time with my partner.

- We find it easy to think of activities to do together.

- I am very satisfied with how we talk to each other.

- We always try to do something nice for each other (without looking for thanks).

- We are creative in how we handle our differences.

- Making joint financial decisions is not difficult.

- We are both equally willing to make adjustments in our relationship.

- I can share feelings and ideas with my partner during disagreements.

- My partner understands my opinions and ideas.

- My partner is my best friend.

- My partner does not try to fix me. We agree it is my job to fix me.

Likewise, the man often has a shallow relationship with his children. Coming out of isolation by sharing time with his children, and beginning to get to know them as precious human beings, contrary to what he experienced during his childhood, changes the dynamic of isolation in the family.

Recovery is not a passive sport

Kerry's story

One day a week Kerry worked from his home office. It was toxic for him to be alone. As part of his acting-out ritual, he looked forward to acting out in the secrecy and comfort of his home office. He would begin the day by addressing work subjects, but would quickly turn to sexually stimulating images on the internet. Kerry knew he needed to change his environment if he wanted to change his acting-out behavior. An alternative for him was to work from a remote site away from his home. When he took positive action to change his environment, he did not act out.

Kerry came to group therapy week after week. While he said he tried, it was difficult for him to make a permanent commitment to not work from his home office when he was alone. He continually talked about other steps he could take, but he was unwilling to take definitive action to reject his addiction.

Addictive behavior will not go away just by attending therapy, Twelve Step meetings, and prayer. The addicted man must formulate a positive plan to change his lifestyle, avoid environmental triggers, and commit to do what is necessary to change the addictive dance.

As the man's spouse or significant other, your understanding and support is part of the man's program. Be willing to listen, but not act as his therapist or accountability partner. Loving listening is very powerful. It is a true act of love. In addition, as noted in chapter 6, this can be an ideal time for you to grow in wisdom by attending self-help groups or participating in your own therapy. (See Appendix E for a list of programs for you.)

Multiple layers of acting-out behavior

Rarely does a man switch off all of his sexually addictive behaviors at one time. Giving up sexual behaviors is often done in stages or layers.

The first layer he will shed is the overt sexual behavior that he believes society rejects. For example, many men find it easier to give up frequenting massage parlors, soliciting prostitutes, engaging in voyeurism, pursuing extra-marital affairs, and participating in other sexually egregious behaviors than to give up pornography and masturbation.

At the second layer, men often address private behavior that is unacceptable at the workplace. Pornography on the internet is a prime example. Most men consider, contrary to reality, that the internet is a private place. Just ask a man who has lost his job because his employer has discovered his use of pornography in the workplace. He unrealistically believed he was in a private space when accessing the internet at work.

The next layer is pornography on the home computer. While the draw to find more sensuous images may continue for some time, a man finally realizes that pornography and masturbation are as toxic as other acting-out behaviors and recovery means rejection of all illicit sexual behaviors.

The last layer he will address is his sexual prism. Sexual addiction is more than just acting-out behavior. At the core of sexual addiction is how a man thinks and perceives the world. The man engages in sexual thinking and fantasies on a daily basis. As noted in Chapter 1, he sees the world through a sexual prism. For example, when he opens a magazine that contains images of men, women, and sometimes children, he will view the images through his sexual prism. If his fetish is women with large breasts, he will check each image against his internal standard. Virtually everything in his world gets processed through his sexual prism. A man who has long given up physically acting-out may still have an active sexual prism. A man who has given up pornography and masturbation may still engage in sexual thinking and fantasy.

Giving up his sexual thinking, fantasy, and prism is perhaps his greatest challenge. He has processed images unconsciously for their sexual content for years, going back into childhood. To be able to pick up a magazine or to watch TV without dwelling on body parts requires a very high level commitment. It may take years for him to work through this layer. For the sexually addicted man, temptation is life-long. What changes is his ability to reject temptation in the present moment. As he invests in sexual sobriety, he gains a commitment not go back to the pain of acting out, and thus is better able to reject all his previous physical acting out behaviors in addition to his sexual prism.

Therapy

It is common to hear a sexually addicted man say, "I don't need therapy, all I have to do is try harder and pray more." He may believe he has his problem under control after a short period of sexual sobriety. Likely he is in denial of the seriousness of his problem and the reason why he is a sexually addicted man.

The nature of compulsivity is the lack of control over one's behavior. The answer for most lies in changing one's life style to address the underlying reasons why addiction is in control. A trained counselor/therapist is in the best position to help a man begin his life-changing journey.

In addition to individual therapy, group therapy is a powerful tool to help sexually addicted men begin to shed the shame of addictive behavior. Group therapy helps men work through their shame and fears. For each man, one of his greatest fears is how he will cope when he gives up his best friend—his sexual addiction. In a group setting men are at different levels of sobriety. Hearing other men's stories serves to enlighten and provide hope.

An essential component of the recovery journey is participation in a Twelve Step program. While individual and group therapy are facilitated by a trained therapist, Twelve Step programs are peer administered. Twelve Step programs have important tasks:

- Benefit from strength. Provide a forum for men and women to talk about their struggle with a common demon—to gather strength from each other.

- Break isolation. Members connect through sharing strengths, hopes, and experiences.

- Foster a learning forum. Personal stories reveal that others think, feel, and behave in similar ways.

- Gather support. Members divulge unhealthy behaviors, and grow into healthy, caring adults who support each other's growth.

- Foster sobriety. Group accountability is a motivator for achieving sobriety.

  A powerful adjunct to Twelve Step meetings are sponsors or accountability partners who are available for frequent contact, encouragement, and accountability. Perhaps the greatest goal is to provide a healing context of working through the Twelve Steps. The Twelve Step programs are time tested and allow the sexually addicted man to continue his journey through time, long after therapy has ended. (For more information on therapy and Twelve Step groups, see Appendix E.)

What can a woman do?

Subsequent to discovering your partner's acting-out sexual behavior, you may wish to consider some or all of the following:

- Insist your partner enter into sexual addiction therapy. You may wish to add a consequence if he does not. (If this is codependent behavior, so be it! This condition is for your health and sanity.)

- Focus on your own recovery. Attend support group programs or engage in individual therapy. Support groups for spouses, or significant others, of addicted men provide information about sexual addiction and boundaries that are important to individual and marital growth. They also provide relationships with other women who are in similar circumstances. During your worst nightmare it is important to know you are not alone.

- Read books on sexual addiction to obtain more insight into this addiction.

- Examine how codependency has governed your marriage relationship. Identify changes you wish to make. It is suggested you do this with the help of a therapist who can guide you through an understanding of the underlying factors that foster codependency.

- Keep the relationship with your partner civil. Don't make decisions with long-term consequences at this time. If you are inclined, be available to listen to your partner's newly gained insights from therapy. Don't play the role of his therapist; just listen.

- Foster non-sexual friendship. Engage in multiple weekly forty-point benchmark activities with your partner.

- Ultimately, marital therapy is part of the recovery journey. Sexual addiction devastates trust and dreams. It may not be possible to recreate old dreams, but it is essential to formulate new shared dreams.

**A marriage based on full confidence, based on complete
and unqualified frankness on both sides;
they are not keeping anything back;
there's no deception underneath it all.
If I might so put it, it's an agreement
for the mutual forgiveness of sin.**

Henrik Ibsen

Chapter Nine

Putting it all Together

We have covered much material in this book. It may be difficult to see the relationship between the various concepts. You may even feel discouraged. Perhaps two more stories will present how two high profile people experienced sexual addiction and subsequently progressed to healing and recovery.

Dr. Mark Laaser, Debbie Laaser (Mark's spouse), Dr. Patrick Carnes, and Marnie C. Ferree appeared February 22, 2004 on Dateline to tell the *Sex Addiction Story*.

Dr. Laaser and Marnie Ferree shared how sex addiction took over their lives. The following stories are from an article by Keith Morrison (2004), *Battling Sex Addiction*, which was based on the Dateline program. See if you can pick out the elements of sexual addiction presented in earlier chapters of this book. A check list follows the stories.

Mark's and Debbie's story

Mark is Rev. Dr. Mark Laaser. According to his web site, Mark Laaser is an internationally known author and speaker. His first book, Faithful and True, was the first Christian book to address the issue of sexual addiction. He has since written six other books including Talking to Your Kids About Sex, and his most recent, The Pornography Trap (with Dr. Ralph Earle). Dr. Laaser has counseled hundreds of sex addicts and their families, consulted with numerous churches, developed treatment programs for a variety of hospitals, and has conducted workshops and seminars worldwide.

Dr. Laaser currently serves as director of the Institute for Healthy Sexuality of the American Association of Christian Counselors, and as executive director of Faithful and True Ministries.

Dr. Laaser holds a PhD in Religion and Psychology from the University of Iowa, a Master of Divinity from Princeton Theological Seminary, and a Bachelors degree in Religion and Philosophy from Augustana College in Rock Island, Illinois. He currently resides in Minnesota with his wife Debbie. They have three grown children: Sarah, Jonathan and Benjamin. Laaser, M. (2012)

Debbie Laaser holds her MA in Marriage and Family Therapy from the Alder Graduate School. She works with her husband, Mark, to provide support for women and counseling couples at their counseling center. She authored Shattered Vows *and was the co-author with Mark of* The Seven Desires of Every Heart. Laaser, D. (2012)

Now Mark and Debbie's story:

(Except for some minor changes, the following text without quotes are the words of Keith Morrison.)

"There was that selfish needy, lonely, angry part of myself that didn't want to stop and saw that sex was my solution to other things," says Mark. He seemed to have an insatiable need for secret sex. To anyone who knew him, it would have seemed incomprehensible. He was married with children, a minister and counselor, an icon of respect. But that wasn't enough. Mark says, early on he felt an emptiness, a loneliness that sex seemed to fill.

"It was just an excitement, a raw excitement—kind of like what a drug addict would describe," says Mark. "It was just a high."

It was a high Mark started experiencing at a young age. When he was 11, he says he discovered pictures, what we'd call soft porn now. "And some of that is not abnormal for a person seeing that for the first time. Of course when it becomes abnormal is how preoccupied you get with it. And then also for me, I started crossing moral boundaries almost right away . . . Stealing magazines—and I'm a preacher's kid, a minister's son. So I knew that stealing was bad. But I was willing to go ahead with it because the high was so fantastic of what I was experiencing."

In high school, Mark hoped his behavior might stop when he met Debbie, the girl he thought could change him.

"There was a part of myself that she just didn't know because I wasn't revealing it to her or anybody for that matter. He wasn't revealing that he was now doing more than looking at magazines. He was watching porn videos and masturbating daily. Debbie, unaware of Mark's double life, trusted him and they got married. Mark hoped that married life would bring an end to a life pre-occupied by sex.

"All this crazy stuff in the past, that will be over now. I'm getting married. I'll have a regular sexual partner and so forth," he reasoned. "But I was amazed early on, even in the first year of marriage, that my temptation to masturbate and look at pornography returned rather quickly."

A lot of people think human beings are preoccupied by sex a lot of time, so what would be so unusual about your feeling? "The part that was unusual was where my mind tended to go with it," says Mark. "I wanted to experience it. I wanted to act it out. Eventually I had a lot of preoccupation with planning or doing or thinking what it would be like."

Mark soon was no longer planning, but doing, paying monthly visits to massage parlors, having sex with so-called "masseuses," all the while hiding it from Debbie, whom Mark says, he still loved deeply.

"I was always completely attracted to her. There was just something so much deeper in me that cannot be satisfied by sex."

He says something deeply emotional was missing, and he wondered why he didn't just stop. "Probably a million times over the course of my acting-out history."

Mark was building toward behavior he would never have thought was possible for him.

He had degrees in religion and divinity, had attended seminary school, was a deeply committed Christian who by this time was an ordained minister. "There was that good side. There was that moral side. There was that caring side." And yet, he'd escape, furtive and guilty, to feed his sexual addiction. At the same time, he was working on getting his PhD in, of all things, psychology.

"Now I'm the Reverend Dr. Laaser. And there are people that are going to be attracted to that and I actually wound up becoming sexual with some of my clients at that time . . . It happened multiple times over a 10-year period . . . [I was] frightened, incredibly frightened . . . I think for years I felt totally worthless. I can't describe to you the times I would sit in church, even preaching on a Sunday morning, thinking God's grace was for everybody else but certainly not for me."

Mark was preaching redemption, but for him, redemption might be more difficult. He betrayed parishioners, colleagues, and clients. It was a trust about to be shattered.

"One of the people I was involved in had reported that—yes, the very thing I was afraid of actually happened. Eight very angry people called me in, canceled my appointments for that day." He says he didn't even realize what they knew, "until the first one opened his mouth and started talking. Then it all came crashing in on me."

His colleagues at the center where he was a counselor angrily confronted and fired him. They would help him get treatment for his sexual misbehavior, but first, they said, he had to tell his wife Debbie, everything.

"I was totally blind sided," says Debbie. "I had no idea that this man I had been living with for 15 years—married to for 15 years—could possibly have been doing all these things. And I'll never forget the look on Mark's face. Actually he was sitting in a chair across from me and I guess today what I know is broken-ness in a person . . . I think there were times truthfully when I questioned whether I would stay. There were times I know when I felt so extremely sad, that I wasn't sure we would ever be able to have happiness in our life again."

And then in the midst of all that pain, her husband felt something else. "This pent up secret that is now over 30 years old is now all of a sudden out of the bag. I don't have to protect the secret anymore. So I think mixed up with fear, sadness and confusion there was a sense of relief."

He has been in recovery for over a decade. He say's it's a continuing process. After his sexual misbehavior was exposed, Mark entered a sex addiction treatment center for a month, where he received psychotherapy called Faithful and True Ministries. He still occasionally goes for counseling and relies on the support of those around him—like Debbie—who stayed by his side through it all.

"I never had these real feelings of just running and leaving," says Debbie. "I wasn't aware that running would solve anything necessarily."

Their relationship eventually strengthened. They dealt with some of the loneliness Mark felt and both found comfort in their religious faith.

"Now that Debbie and I are more spiritually intimate, sex in our relationship is totally satisfying," says Mark.

His work has also helped him. He is again counseling others—including men with problems like his

Marnie's story

Marnie C. Ferree is a licensed marriage and family therapist employed with the Woodmont Hills Church in Nashville, Tennessee, which is the sponsoring organization for Bethesda Workshops. She has a national reputation as a

leader in the field of sexual addiction, particularly as it presents in women. In 1997, Marnie established a workshop program for female sex addicts that was the first of its kind in the country and today draws participants from across the United States and Canada. She has directed Bethesda Workshops since 2000. Previously, Marnie provided counseling for sexual recovery (both from sexual abuse and sexual addiction) through the Woodmont Hills Counseling Center, a sister ministry at the church. Marnie is a frequent lecturer at professional and recovery conferences, churches, and schools. She also consults with Christian organizations and churches about sexual integrity, especially in cases where a leader has fallen into sexual sin.

Marnie's book about female sexual addiction, "No Stones: Women Redeemed from Sexual Shame," is the first Christian book on the subject by a woman personally in recovery. No Stones has been widely acclaimed as a pioneering work and is considered the standard in the field. Her second book is "L.I.F.E. Guide for Women," a workbook for female sex addicts.

Marnie and her husband David have been married since 1981 and are parents of a young adult son, married daughter and grandparents of an infant grandson. (Ferree, 2012)

Now Marnie's story:

(Except for some minor changes, the following text without quotes are the words of Keith Morrison.)

"I was wracked with shame and tried time and time again to stop," says Marnie.

Like Mark, she knows what it's like to be out of control. For Marnie, it wasn't so much about sex itself, but about the relationships she thought she could have by engaging in sex with acquaintances and friends.

"The sexual part was pleasurable and it was a nice by product for me but that wasn't the most important thing. I was trying to get non sexual needs met sexually and that was the only way I knew how to meet those needs."

As a child, Marnie was sexually abused by a family friend, a not uncommon precursor to later addiction. Her promiscuity lasted from her teen years through two marriages, with numerous affairs. She felt an emotional void she says that sex filled—at least initially.

"At the time there is an incredible adrenaline rush. It's a connection that I found I couldn't replicate anywhere else. But immediately after that experience is over, I mean driving back home, there is this incredible letdown and you're just in a wash of shame."

That shame that worsened after Marnie was diagnosed with cervical cancer. The cause, she was told, was a sexually transmitted disease.

"That was the lowest point. I experienced three surgeries in a year as treatment of that cervical cancer. Had a major hemorrhaging after one of those surgeries. I mean my life was literally in danger and I found still that I could not stop."

She was sick, married, a mother, and yet none of those things could make her change, even though she was horrified by what she was doing.

"It's about feeling rotten. I want to feel better. What way am I going through a ritual to feel better? I'm connecting with someone; I'm going to act out sexually. I feel horrible after that and the whole cycle starts over again."

Marnie was desperate. Sex with her husband was not enough, and she believed the only way to stop having sex outside her marriage, was to end her life. "I had really strong suicidal thoughts. But I knew I couldn't keep on living but I was too afraid to die."

"I've sometimes gone home with people I'm not even that attracted to and yet I feel like if I don't have sex with them it's just the most horrible feeling." Marnie thought sex was her solution to painful feelings, but it was a solution that was not working.

After years of failing to will herself to stop having sex with acquaintances, she was ready to take her own life. And then, at last, she confided in someone. "I picked up the phone and called a dear friend and poured out this awful saga of my life and said I need help."

She did get help. A therapist helped her learn to deal with the childhood sexual abuse that contributed to her many affairs. Her second marriage survived and is, she says, better. She was surprised to find she wasn't alone.

About a third of sex addicts are female, which is why, to do something to help other women, she went back to school to get a degree in counseling. "I didn't choose sex addiction. Sex addiction chose me and this field chose me. Women are afraid to talk about it. We're afraid of being labeled as whores. It's kind of guys will be guys, men will be men. But for a woman to be out of control in her sexual behavior there is just a whole other level of shame."

What did you find in these stories?

Dr. Mark Laaser, Debbie Laaser (Mark's spouse), and Marnie Ferree showed courage in sharing their stories on Dateline. They provide a broad spectrum of characteristics found in sexual addiction. Your challenge is to read their stories carefully and to see if you have found the characteristics listed below:

- The power of sexual addiction and overcoming the desire to continue to act out.

- Secret sex.

- Addiction that began in childhood.

- The expectation that marriage would end the temptation to act out.

- The preoccupation with planning and time to act out.

- Hiding behind the mask of respectability and leading a dual life.

- Impact on relationship with God.

- Denial.

- Unmanageability of acting-out behavior.

- Out of control life.

- Abused as a child.

- Shame of acting out.

- Blind to consequences.

- Acting-out cycle.

- Medicating pain.

- Addiction based on relationship expectations.

- Suicidal thoughts.

- Disclosing secrets as the first step to healing.

- Decision to change.

- A new outcome.

- Healing.

Paul Becker, LPC

Summary

For the wife or significant other who is dealing with a sexually impacted partner in the open for the first time, the complexity of the addiction can be overwhelming. (Books listed in the Appendix D will provide more information, if you desire.)

Please remember, your partner did not become sexually addicted overnight, and he will not become totally sober overnight. Both Bradshaw and Carnes believe that the recovery journey takes years. (Carnes, 1991, Bradshaw, 1988)

An important question for many women is: should I stay or should I leave my partner? Unfortunately, the answer is not a simple yes or no. As Dr.Mark Laaser witnessed, his wife Debbie stayed with him. The recovery has fostered a new sense of life for both of them.

On the other hand, Marnie Ferree's first husband did not stay with her. At the time of her divorce from her first husband, she was not ready for an addiction-free relationship.

One of the tenets of marriage therapy is: when a marriage is in difficulty, the partners are well advised to solve their relationship problems in their present environment because, if they don't, they will repeat the same problems in their next relationship. While you did not in any manner cause your partner's addictive behavior, your personality type and the wounds you suffered while growing up contributed to the dynamics of the marriage. In marriages that include a sexually addicted man, the spouse is often advised to enter therapy to address her own issues.

Generally, therapy for the family which includes a sexually addicted man is not over until the couple participates in marriage therapy. Overcoming codependency in the marriage is a key to long-term recovery.

Appendix A

Unwanted Sexual Behaviors Found
in the DSM-IV-TR

The bible of definitions for counselors and therapists is the *Diagnostic and Statistical Manual of Mental Disorders, DSM IV* for short. The *DSM IV* satisfies the need to classify mental disorders, to agree on common definitions, to offer diagnostic assistance to mental health specialists, to codify insurance processing, and to carry out statistical analysis. It is the product of much research and study and represents the American Psychiatric Association's guidance to the mental health community at large.

The *DSM IV* classifies only a small proportion of what are considered unwanted sexual behaviors. But it is a good place to start. It defines unwanted sexual behaviors as paraphilias. (American Psychiatric Association, 2000) All paraphilias, according to the *DSM IV*, are characterized by reoccurring, intense sexual urges, sexual fantasies, or behaviors. Such fantasies, sexual urges, or behaviors must occur over at least a six-month period of time. They must also cause significant stress or impair one's social, occupational, or everyday functioning for a diagnosis to be made. There is also a sense of distress within these individuals. Typically, one recognizes the symptoms as negatively impacting their lives but believes they are unable to control them.

Paraphilias included in the *DSM-IV-TR* are:

- **Exhibitionism** involves the surprise exposure of one's genitals to a stranger. Exposure may coincide with masturbation and a fantasy expectation that the stranger will become sexually aroused.

- **Fetishism** involves the use of nonliving objects, for example, a woman's undergarments, or other worn apparel, to achieve a state of arousal. The man frequently masturbates while holding, rubbing, or smelling the apparel. He may ask his sexual partner to wear the apparel during sexual encounters. The fetish is either preferred or required for sexual excitement.

- **Frotteurism** involves touching and rubbing one's genitals against a non-consenting person. The behavior generally occurs in crowded places to avoid arrest. The behavior may also involve fondling. During the act the person usually fantasizes an exclusive, caring relationship with the victim.

- **Pedophilia** is characterized by sexual activity with a child, usually age 13 or younger, or in the case of an adolescent, a child five years younger than the pedophile.

- **Masochism** involves the act of being humiliated, beaten, bound, or otherwise made to suffer to enhance or achieve sexual excitement. In some cases the act is limited to a fantasy of being raped while being held or bound by others so that there is no possibility of escape. Sexual Masochism may involve a wide range of devices to achieve the desired effect, including some that may cause death.

- **Sadism** involves an act in which the individual derives sexual excitement from the psychological or physical suffering, including humiliation, of the victim. The partner may or may not be consenting. Sadism may involve a wide range of behaviors and devices to achieve the desired effect.

- **Transvestic fetishism** involves heterosexual males who dress in female clothes (cross-dressing) to produce or enhance sexual arousal, usually without a real partner, but with the fantasy that they are the female partner. Women's garments are arousing primarily as symbols of the individual's femininity.

- **Voyeurism** involves observing an unknowing and non-consenting person, usually a stranger, who is naked or in the process of becoming unclothed and/or engaging in sexual activity. The act of looking (peeping) is intended to produce sexual excitement and is usually accompanied by self-masturbation. Fantasies from such acts are used to fuel future masturbation.

Unwanted Sexual Behaviors NOT Found in DSM-IV-TR

The following unwanted sexual behaviors are not included in the *DSM-IV-TR* but may likewise result in significant stress or impair one's social, occupational or everyday functioning.

- **Extra-marital affairs** involve single or multiple sexual relationships with partners outside the marriage that cause significant stress to the marriage relationship. Men often justify an affair because of a perception of unfulfilled expectations within the marriage. Swinging and wife swapping are aberrant forms of extramarital affairs that include the participation of both marriage partners.

- **Multiple or anonymous partners** often involve homosexual relationships— frequently anonymous, situational, and intended to provide sexual experience. Homosexual encounters also may be habitual since they are repeated time and again with new partners. They are particularly dangerous to the parties if practiced without the protection of a condom because participants are exposed to venereal disease and/or HIV.

- **Prostitution** involves the solicitation and procurement of various types of sexual behavior from male or female escorts or prostitutes.

- **Sexual massage** involves the solicitation and procurement of sex, most often, oral sex or masturbation, from a male or female who provides massages. In most cases those who seek such services engage in other unwanted sexual behaviors.

- **Sexual anorexia** involves an obsessive state in which the physical, mental, and emotional tasks of avoiding sex dominate one's life. Preoccupation with the avoidance of sex may be used to mask or avoid one's life problems. The obsession can then become a way to cope with all stress and all life difficulties.

Compulsive sexual behaviors

Our society judges some sexual behaviors as reasonably normal. Among men, little stigma is attached to them. The concepts "every male does it" or "it doesn't hurt anyone" or similar thinking is used to justify the behavior. What changes a behavior from acceptable to unacceptable is compulsivity, that is, it is engaged in excessively; becomes time consuming; interferes with a person's daily routine, work, or social functioning; continues despite no longer being pleasurable or gratifying; places the individual at risk of physical harm; or has legal or personal consequences and leads to financial debt. Examples include:

- **Masturbation** involves sexual self-stimulation, most commonly by touching, stroking, or massaging the penis, clitoris, or vagina until orgasm is achieved. Masturbation is the most common form of sexual addiction.

- **Pornography** is any material that depicts or describes sexual function for the purpose of stimulating sexual arousal upon the part of the consumer.

- **Cybersex** has as its common elements the use of a computer, internet access, expected anonymity, and sexually provocative material to generate arousal followed most often by masturbation. Multiple venues such as visual images of real or graphic generated persons, interactive sex through a web cam, chat rooms, and e-mail exist. Cybersex is increasing at a high rate.

- **Phone Sex** has as its common element the use of a phone to talk or listen to a provocative repertoire to generate arousal followed, most often, by masturbation.

Appendix B

Sex Addiction Cycle

Men who deal with unwanted sexual behavior find themselves repeating a cycle of thinking and events called a "sex addiction cycle."

In *Out of the Shadows,* (1994) and again in *Contrary to Love,* (1989) Carnes writes eloquently about the sex addiction cycle. This section is an adaptation of his concept.

One of the principle characteristics of addiction is that the act is repetitive to the point in which the addict becomes powerless to change the outcome. Each time he goes through the acting out process he completes a cycle. In short, there is a beginning thought process, a build up, the act, the let down (guilt, grief and pledges to do better, and self justification), and a return to the beginning.

Below are the sequential steps or phases experienced by a sexually addicted person from the addict's point of view. Within each phase the addict will engage in thinking described in one or more of the subtitles under each phase. The time an addict takes to repeat the cycle can vary from minutes to months. A compulsive masturbator may act out five or more times a day, whereas a man involved in affairs may only act out when circumstances permit.

Initial Phase—Life Condition

Victim posture. In my belief system, I am a victim in this world and not responsible for my behavior. In a new situation, I look for ways I will be hurt. I may not even know that I look to be a victim. I have poor boundaries—people take advantage of me.

Low-grade depression. Life for me is an existence; I often think life is passing me by. Except when acting out, I am rarely happy and I never feel joy.

Anticipated rejection. I create situations in which someone else can reject me. I hold people at a distance. I can't let people know my real self—I know they will not love me.

Social isolation. I live behind a mask of respectability but underneath my mask is my real self. I simply cannot let anyone in. If I did, they would see that I am really a bad person. I have few or no real friends. No one really knows who I am.

Emotional isolation. I am neither in touch with my own feelings nor with other people's feelings. I don't understand that I hurt others. I don't understand my own feelings. For me, intimacy means sex.

Phase Two—Reaction to Life Condition

Escapism. Living life is just too boring or I feel like life is just one painful experience after another. I need to find ways of relieving my bad feelings.

Need-fulfilling fantasy. I don't know how to cope, thus I daydream of a better life. I use fantasy to get temporary relief.

Sexual fantasy. I use sexual fantasies or visual sexual stimulation to escape my pain. My next act is often the subject of my fantasies and my sexual thinking. My fantasy is my best friend—we see each other a lot.

Sexual materials. I maintain a well-used stash of pornographic magazines and movies, Web sites, and sex toys. Whenever I feel lonely, tired, or angry, my stash is nearby to raise my mood.

Phase Three—Acting out

Acting-out ritual. I mentally begin a ritual that leads to acting out. At times I play games with myself. As examples, I tell myself I will just go a little way but not all the way—but go all the way. I go to the internet to check mail but not porn—but end up at a porn site.

Acting out. Sex is my most important need. I act out sexually even when I don't want to.

Phase Four—Reconciliation

Transitory guilt. I feel sorry and ashamed of myself. I fear being caught. My focus is on what is going to happen to me. I am unaware of how I hurt my family. My feeling of guilt is short-lived.

Reconstruction. I present outwardly that I am a good guy. I seek forgiveness at church. I am never going to do it again. I am going to make it right. I conceal my act.

Mistaken beliefs. I didn't hurt anybody. I deserve some pleasure in life.

Thinking errors. I can control it if I want to. I don't need any help. What do they know about my problem?

Once completed, the addict returns to the initial phase and begins the cycle anew.

Acting-Out Ritual

Every addict repeats an acting-out ritual before acting out. "The rituals contain a set of well-rehearsed cues which trigger arousal." (Carnes, 1983)

> The ritual seems magically to bring order out of chaos. Think of it as a dance—certain steps, certain sounds, ceremony, rhythm, special artifacts—which can be very elaborate but have one purpose: to put addicts into another world so they can escape the conditions of real life over which they think they have no control. Fantasy is compounded by delusion at this point; the mood-altered state is a 'world' in which the addicts no longer care about control in the same way. Sexual obsession is pursued to its peak regardless of risk, harm, or other consequences. There is only one kind of control that matters now—control of sexual pleasure. Once they start dancing, they rarely, if ever, can stop on their own. (Carnes, 1989)

Rituals are often connected to places, things, or activities. For example, Mason knew the location of all the massage parlors in his city. He would cruise the neighborhoods nearby, tell himself he was not going near a massage parlor, but found himself repeatedly parking nearby. For others, the rituals may include visiting parks, swimming pools, shopping malls, restrooms, movie theaters, porn shops, peepshows, or other locations that are part of the pattern used by the addict to set the stage for acting out. The TV remote is a curse for many a man. Channel flipping is like a gun with one round in the chamber. Sooner or later a channel will provide the visual stimulation needed to activate the lust pattern.

Men are usually not cognizant of the consistency of their ritualization patterns until they are asked to record the events that lead to an orgasm. They are even more surprised to discover their ritual often begins long before they take any action. Initial steps in the ritual may begin with feelings of Hunger, Anger, Loneliness, and Tiredness, often referred to by the acronym HALT. Since addicted men frequently live in a state of low-grade depression, feelings of being down may trigger a need to alter their mood and thus their ritual.

Sexually addicted men have one or more acting-out rituals. Once the addict has passed through the initial steps of his ritual, he hits a slippery slope. Picture a ski slope. While at the bottom of the slope, he still has choices. The mind of the addict doesn't correlate riding the chairlift with acting out, so he stands in line and rides to the top of the slope. While standing at the top, he can convince himself that a leisurely ride will not result in acting out but he must be careful not to gain too much speed or to hit a patch of ice that will render him out of control. While cruising through long, sweeping turns, feeling comfortable, the mind of the addict wants to go a little faster, and a little faster after that. Suddenly the addict is barreling down the slippery slope toward certain sexual acting out and he doesn't understand why. The mind of the addict isn't willing to consider all the decisions that brought him to the speed and direction he is currently taking. Instead, he blames a patch of ice or the slope itself. The slippery slope of his addiction begins when he sees the chairlift, not when his speed and direction don't allow him to stop.

Appendix C

Family Environment and Structure

Most sexually addicted men come from a family environment that did not meet their childhood need for affection or emotional support. Often children who live in dysfunctional families feel a sense of abandonment by their parents. The parents simply were not there for the child in a way that led to feelings of self-confidence and love. The child felt isolated from his parents and siblings.

The family was usually either rigid or chaotic. If the family was rigid, the child thought that he had to measure up to his parents' expectations of him or he may have concluded that he was not a worthy human being. Family rules were conveyed explicitly, often by yelling, critical nagging, or body language. Body language in a rigid family may include the deep sigh, a frown, abruptly disconnected conversation, or the look that could kill. In either mode, the child receives the message that he is deficient. A rigid family is often performance-based. That is, for the child to be loved, he has to perform. Getting good grades, doing well in sports, and having a physically fit body are some examples of conditional love. The child frequently thinks that it is not possible for him to perform in the way his parents require. The old adage, "children are to be seen and not heard," is characteristic of a rigid family. The family is run by a system of rules. Punishment for not abiding the rules of behavior brings parental scorn.

In his book, *Facing the Shadow*, Carnes (2001) says:

> "Sex addicts also tend to come from rigid, authoritarian families. These are families in which all issues and problems are black and white. Little is negotiable and there is only one way to do things. Success in the family means doing what the parents want to such an extent that children give up being who they are. Normal child development does not happen. By the time children enter adolescence, they have few options. One is to become rebellious. The other is to develop a secret life about which the family knows nothing. Both positions distort reality. Both result in a distrust of authority and a poor sense of self.
>
> If the family's rigidity is also sex negative (that is, children are taught that sex is dirty, sinful, bad, or nasty), sex becomes exaggerated or hidden. Worse yet, the forbidden can become the object of obsession. Or all of the above may happen. The worst-case scenario happens when the child finds out that parents are not living up to their sexual standards. For example, if the parents

preach against sexual promiscuity but one or both chronically have affairs, this teaches the acceptability of sexual duplicity. The norm is to deceive others and to pretend that what is true is not true."

The chaotic family is on the opposite end of the spectrum. A child in a chaotic family thinks he has no thoughts that are his own. His parents are always penetrating the boundaries of his world. The child has no space he can call his own. In a chaotic situation the family name is of paramount importance. It is the job of all family members to look good to the neighbors. If a member of the family fails, it is the job of the family to close ranks and protect the wounded member.

In both a rigid and a chaotic family, the child ends up feeling the same. He is not loved for who he is as a human being. Such children feel isolated and seek other avenues to express themselves. For some it becomes sex even though sex is often considered bad or dirty and is rarely talked about.

When a child feels isolated and detached from his parents, he is unable to go to them with confidence that they will love him when something bad has happened. For most young children who are exposed to age-inappropriate behavior or material, instinct tells them that something bad has happened. Their fear of parental discovery discourages them away from the very healing that comes from parental intervention.

This is the very time that a child needs his parents most. It is critical that parents are called upon to explain to the child that his exposure to age-inappropriate behavior or material was not his fault, and as a child, he could not be responsible. Parental guidance is needed to explain that the normal body reaction to sexual material—arousal—is not bad. It is normal at the proper time and circumstances. A traumatized child needs to know that he is loved unconditionally and that this bad event does not change his parents' love.

When a child believes he cannot trust his parents to love him at the time of exposure to age-inappropriate behavior or material, he withdraws into himself and becomes even more isolated. He now has a huge troubling secret that he believes he cannot share. Many children even begin to blame themselves for the event, when all the logical signs point elsewhere. The child is often permanently damaged.

Appendix D

Publications

Books by Dr. Patrick Carnes

Carnes, P. (1997). The Betrayal Bond: Breaking Free of Exploitive Relationships. Deerfield Beach, FL: Health Communications.

> This book presents an in-depth study of exploitive relationships: why they form, who is most susceptible, and how they become so powerful. It explains to readers how to recognize when traumatic bonding has occurred and provides a checklist so they can examine their own relationships. Included are steps readers can take to safely extricate themselves or their loved ones from these situations.

Carnes, P. (2001). Facing the Shadow: Starting Sexual and Relationship Recovery. Carefree, AZ: Gentle Path Press.

> This workbook is designed as a companion to *Out of the Shadows*, *Don't Call It Love*, and *Sexual Anorexia*. It includes exercises to help work through such subjects as denial, understanding the addictive cycle, and identifying compulsive behaviors.

Carnes, P. (1994). A Gentle Path Through the 12 Steps. Center City, MN: Hazelden.

> This book provides exercises, inventories, and guided reflections for those who face the daily challenge of attaining or maintaining an addiction-free lifestyle.

Carnes, P. (1992). Don't Call It Love: Recovery From Sexual Addiction. New York, NY: Bantam

> This book is based on the testimony of more than one thousand recovering sexual addicts in the first major scientific study of the disorder. It includes findings of Dr. Carnes's research and advice from the addicts and co-addicts as they work to overcome their compulsive behavior. This book helps the reader to better understand all addictions, their causes, and the difficult path to recovery.

Carnes, P. (1994). Contrary to Love: Helping the Sexual Addict. Center City, MN: Hazelden

> This book provides mental health professionals with a resource for understanding and helping sexual addicts. Subjects outlined include stages and progression of the illness, family structures, boundaries, assessment, and intervention.

Carnes, P. (2001). Out of the Shadows: Understanding Sexual Addiction. (Rev. 3rd ed.). Center City, MN: Hazelden.

> This book, the first to describe sexual addiction, is the standard for recognizing and overcoming this destructive behavior. It outlines how to identify a sexual addict, recognize the way others may unwittingly become complicit or codependent, and change the patterns that support the addiction.

Carnes, P., Lasser, D., & Lasser, M. (2000). Open Hearts: Renewing Relationships with Recovery, Romance and Reality. Carefree, AZ: Gentle Path Press.

> This book will guide the reader along a pathway of self-assessment, discovery, and fulfillment. Proven techniques from Recovering Couples Anonymous help couples overcome anger, resentment, and dysfunctional patterns, thus allowing them to enjoy the intimate, fulfilling relationship they long for. It is a book a couple does together. It takes techniques Carnes and Laaser developed in their psychotherapy practices and weaves them into a series of individual and joint exercises. It looks at tough issues: shame, anger, money, betrayal, sex, parenting. It encourages fun like drawing up a family motto, expressing spirituality together, and taking gentleness breaks.

Carnes, P., Delmonico, D. & Griffi n, E. (2001). In the Shadows of the Net: Breaking Free of Compulsive Online Sexual Behavior. Center City, MN: Hazelden.

> This book explains how the anonymity of online access, the ability of people to use their computers in private, and the powerful rationalization that virtual interactions are not "real" can combine to entice people to spend hours online, sacrificing real relationships and increasing their sense of loneliness.

> The book provides a Internet Screening Test to help people decide if they have a problem with their use of sexual material on the internet.

Carnes, P., & Adams, K. (2003). The Clinical Management of Sex Addiction. New York, NY: Brunner-Routledge.

> This is the first comprehensive volume of the clinical management of sex addiction. Collecting the work of twenty-eight leaders in this emerging field, the editors provide a long-needed primary text about how to approach

treatment with these challenging patients. The book serves as an introduction for professionals new to the field as well as serving as a useful reference tool. The contributors are pioneers of addiction medicine and sex therapy.

Carnes, P. (2010). Recovery Zone, Volume 1: Making Changes that Last, The Internal Tasks. Carefree, AZ: Gentle Path Press.

This workbook notes that recovery from addiction is a work in progress and that many things must change simultaneously for recovery to work. The book shares strategies for maintaining and nurturing recovery, in the early days and beyond.

Selected articles by Dr. Patrick Carnes

Carnes, P. (1986). Sex addict speaks SIECUS Report, XIV (6).

Carnes, P. (1987, May). Sexual addiction: Implications for spiritual formation. Studies in Formative Spirituality, Journal of Ongoing Formation.

Carnes, P. (1988). Sexually addicted families: Using the Circumplex. Journal of Psychotherapy and the Family.

Carnes, P. (1988, Nov./Dec.). Bars and bordellos: Sexual addiction and chemical dependency. Professional Counselor.

Carnes, P. (1989). Contrary to love: The sex addict. building bridges, creating balance.

Monograph of AAMFT, San Francisco Annual Conference Plenary Presentations.

Carnes, P. (1989, Nov./Dec.). Sexual addiction. Professional Counselor.

Carnes, P. (1990). Sexual addiction. The Incest Perpetrator: A Family Member No One Wants to Treat. Editors: Horton, A.L., Johnson, B.L., Roundy, L.M., Williams, D., Sage Publications.

Carnes, P. (1990, May). Sexual addiction: Progress, criticism, challenges. American Journal of Preventive Psychiatry & Neurology. 2:3.

Carnes, P. (1991, Nov./Dec.). Sexual addiction. The Counselor.

Carnes, P. (1993). Addiction and posttraumatic stress: The convergence of victim's realities. Treating Abuse Today. 3(3), 5-11.

Carnes, P. (1993, May/June). When the issue is sex addiction. Addiction & Recovery.

Carnes, P. (1993, June). Abused children: Addicted adults. Changes.

Carnes, P., Skilling, N., Nonemaker, D., & Delmonico, D. (1993, June). Study of the relationship between childhood abuse and adulthood addictive behavior in a sample of identified sexual addicts. Paper presented at the National Council for Sexual Addictions Conference.

Carnes, P. & Delmonico, D. (1996). Childhood abuse and multiple addictions: Research findings in a sample of self-identified sexual addicts. Sexual Addiction & Compulsivity: The Journal of Treatment and Prevention. 3:3, 258.

Carnes, P. (1998, Feb.). The obsessive shadow. Professional Counselor.

Carnes, P. (1998). Scandal and significance: The problem of being powerful and powerless." Professional Counselor. 13:6, 13.

Carnes, P. (1998). The case for sexual anorexia: An interim report on 144 patients with sexual disorders. Sexual Addiction & Compulsivity: The Journal of Treatment and Prevention. 5:4, 293.

Carnes, P. & Delmonico, D. (1999). Virtual sex addiction: When cybersex becomes the drug of choice. CyberPsychology & Behavior. 2(5), 457-462.

Carnes, P. (1999, Sept./Oct.). Case study: A question of character. Harvard Business Review. 40-41.

Carnes, P. & Schneider, J. (2000, May/June). Recognition and management of addictive sexual disorders: Guide for the primary care clinician. Primary Care Practice. 4:3, 302-318. Lippincott Williams & Wilkins.

Carnes, P. (2000). Sexual addiction and compulsion: Recognition, treatment and recovery. CNS Spectrums. 5:10, 63-72.

Carnes, P. (2000) Eroticized rage and other sexualized feelings. Professional Counselor. 14:2, pp. 12-16, 52-54.

Carnes, P. (2000). Sexual compulsion: Challenge for church leaders. Addiction and Compulsive Behaviors. The National Catholic Bioethics Center: Boston, Massachusetts. 93-112.

Carnes, P. (2001). Cybersex, courtship and escalating arousal: Factors in addictive sexual desire. Sexual Addiction & Compulsivity: The Journal of Treatment and Prevention. 8:1.

Carnes, P. (2001). Sober sex. 12: Life in recovery. Guideposts. 14-15.

Carnes, P. (May 2001). Understanding addictive disorders. Recovery Today. 6:5. Rev 4/01.

Other readings

David Delmonico. D., Griffin, E., and Moriarity, J. (2001). Cybersex Unhooked: A Workbook for Breaking Free of Compulsive Online Sexual Behavior. Carefree, AZ: Gentle Path Press.

> This book helps people understand their cybersex behaviors, and provides concrete exercises that will help them break free from their compulsive online sexual behavior.

Arterburn, S., Stoeker, F., & Yorkey, M. (2000). Every Man's Battle: Winning the War on Sexual Temptation One Victory at a Time. Colorado Springs, CO: WaterBrook Press.

> This book describes the challenge every man faces—the fight every man can win—sexual temptation. From the television to the internet, print media to videos, men are constantly faced with the assault of sensual images. The book denies the perception men are unable to control their thought lives and roving eyes. The book shares the stories of men who have escaped the trap of sexual immorality and presents a practical, detailed plan for any man who desires sexual purity-perfect for men who have fallen in the past, those who want to remain strong today, and all who want to overcome temptation in the future. It includes a section for women, designed to help them understand and support the men they love.

Arterburn, S., Stoeker, F., & Yorkey, M. (2002). Every Man's Battle Workbook: The Path to Sexual Integrity Starts Here. Colorado Springs, CO: WaterBrook Press.

> This book is a practical guide for individuals and men's groups designed to help men win the war on sexual temptation. It is a companion workbook to Every Man's Battle.

Becker, P. (2010). In Search of Recovery: A Christian Man's Guide. Carefree, AZ: Gentle Path Press.

> This book was written for men who find themselves engaged in unwanted sexual behavior or otherwise known as sexually addicted. It offers insights into the nature of sexual addiction; the sexual addiction cycle and acting-out rituals; the role of anger, anxiety, and depressed mood in sexual addiction; and spirituality in recovery. It asks and answers the question: Is there hope I can change my behavior?

Becker, P. (2010) In Search of Recovery Workbook: A Christian Man's Guide. Carefree, AZ: Gentle Path Press.

> This book is a companion workbook to *In Search of Recovery: A Christian Man's Guide*. It provides structured exercise for use in either individual or

group therapy. It offers many useful insights and how to move out of addiction and into a more fulfilling life.

Bradshaw, J. (1988). Bradshaw on: The Family. Deerfield Beach, FL: Health Communications.

> This book focuses on the dynamics of the family, how the rules and attitudes learned while growing up become encoded within each family member. It guides the reader out of dysfunction to wholeness and teaches bad beginnings can be remedied.

Cooper, A. (Ed.). (2001). Sex and the Internet: A Guide for Clinicians. New York, NY: Brunner-Routledge.

> Sex and the Internet is the first professional book on Internet sexuality. This book is a clinician's guide that addresses Internet sexuality by both informing and providing practical and concrete suggestions and directions. The book is compilation of contributions by international experts in the field of sexuality including Patrick Carnes.

Corley, D., & Schneider, J. (2002). Disclosing Secrets: When, to Whom and How Much and to Reveal. Carefree, AZ: Gentle Path Press.

> This book is a guide to revealing sexual addiction secrets to one's spouse and others. The book takes the reader through the painful process of revealing addiction related secrets—what, where, when to tell and who to involve.

Crow, G., Earle R., & Osborn, K. (1989). Lonely All the Time: Recognizing, Understanding and Overcoming Sex Addiction, for Addicts and Codependents. New York, NY: Pocket Books (Div. Of Simon & Schuster).

> This book is a comprehensive, practical approach to recovery for the addict. It explains what sex addiction is and how to recover from sex addiction. The book explores the causes and symptoms of sex addiction. It also includes a practical approach to recovery for the addict and family.

Carnes, S. (Ed) (2008). Mending a Shattered Heart—A Guide for Partners of Sex Addicts. Carefree, AZ: Gentle Path Press.

> This book is for the spouse who needs an answer to the question: Where do I go from here? Many discover their loved one, the one person that they are supposed to trust, has been living a life of lies and deceit because they suffer from a disease—a disease called sex addiction.?

McDaniel, K (2008-2nd ed.). Ready to Heal—Women Facing Love, Sex & Relationship Issues. Carefree, AZ: Gentle Path Press.

Many women experience the pain of an addictive relationship-the kind of relationship that's painful to be in, yet impossible to leave. The book walks the reader through an assessment of how women get into these relationships and a guide to recovery.

Gordon, J. R., & Marlat, G. A. (Eds.). (1985). Relapse Prevention: Maintenance Strategies in the Treatment of Addictive Behaviors. New York, NY: Guilford Publications.

This book analyzes factors that may lead to relapse and offers practical techniques for maintaining treatment gains.

Hendrix, H. (2001). Getting the Love You Want: A Guide for Couples (Rep. ed.). New York, NY: Owl Books.

This book presents relationship skills to help couples replace confrontation and criticism with a healing process of mutual growth and support. It describes the techniques of Imago Relationship Therapy, which combines a number of disciplines—including the behavioral sciences, depth psychology, cognitive therapy, and Gestalt therapy, among others—to create a program to resolve conflict and renew communication and passion.

Hope and Recovery: A Twelve Step Guide for Healing From Compulsive Sexual Behavior. (1987). Minneapolis, MI: CompCare Publishers.

This was one of the first books to comprehensively describe the application of the Twelve Steps of Alcoholics Anonymous to sexual addiction and compulsivity. It also includes a wide range of personal stories in which recovering sexual addicts share their experience, strength, and hope.

Kasl, C. D. (2002). Many Roads, One Journey: Moving Beyond the Twelve Steps. Saint Helens, OR: Perennial Press.

This book, from the author of Women, Sex, and Addiction, is a timely and controversial second look at Twelve Step programs. It is intended to help readers draw on the steps' underlying wisdom and adapting them to their own experiences, beliefs, and sources of strength.

Laaser, M. (2004). Healing the Wounds of Sexual Addiction. Grand Rapids, MI:Zondervan Publishing Company.

This book is written by a former sex addict. It offers help and hope for regaining and maintaining sexual integrity, self-control, and wholesome, biblical sexuality.

Milkman, H., & Sunderwirth, S. (1998). Craving for Ecstasy: How Our Passions Become Addictions and What We Can Do About Them (Rep ed.). San Francisco, CA: Jossey-Bass.

This book describe the variety of addictive ways individuals lose control of their lives while striving for pleasure and escape. Addictive behavior goes beyond the compulsive use of drugs and alcohol. It is possible to become addicted to what may seem a harmless pleasure such as sex, jogging, watching television, and eating. This book explains the biology, chemistry, and psychology of the universal desire for pleasure and escape. For example, it reveals how the brain produces "mind-altering" substances and what the skydiver has in common with the heroin addict. With the use of a self assessment test and a guide for treatment, the book shows what steps one can take to regain control of one's life.

Schaumburg, H. (1997). False Intimacy: Understanding the Struggle of Sexual Addiction (Rev. ed.). Colorado Springs, CO: Navpress Publishing Group.

This book, set in a Christian context, examines the roots behind destructive sexual behaviors and offers realistic direction to those whose lives or ministries have been impacted by sexual addiction.

Schneider, B., & Schneider, J. (2004). Sex Lies and Forgiveness: Couples Speaking Out on Healing from Sex Addiction (3rd ed.). Recovery Resources Press.

In this book, 88 couples talk about how they have coped with the problem of addictive sexual behavior.

Schneider, J. (2001). Back from Betrayal: Recovering from His Affairs (2nd ed.).Recovery Resources Press.

This book provides practical help for women involved with sex addicted men. The second edition is expanded and updated, with a new chapter for men whose partner is a sex addict, and another new chapter on living with a cybersex addict.

Weiss, D. (2000). Steps to Freedom (2nd ed.). Colorado Springs, CO: Discovery Press.

This book follows the tradition of the Twelve Steps from a Christian perspective. It breaks down the various principles to help the reader experience freedom from sex addiction.

Weiss, R. and Schneider, J. (2006). Untangling the Web: Sex, Porn and Fantasy Obsession. New York, NY: Alyson Books.

This book provides personal stories from addicts and their significant others. It is a resource which offers healing strategies for anyone experiencing the negative impact of Internet pornography and sex addiction

Kasl, C. (1990). Women, Sex, and Addiction: A Search for Love and Power. New York, NY: Harper Paperbacks

This book guides women to understand sexual addiction and sexual codependency and to lead them to recovery. Women will learn to experience their sexuality as a source of love and positive power, and sex as an expression that honors the soul as well as the body.

Appendix E

Counseling and Support Programs

Where can help be found?

Help for the sexually addicted man comes in many forms. In this Appendix you will find many venues for help including counseling and Twelve Step programs. All of the material provided has been downloaded from public Web sites.

Individual counseling

Society for the Advancement of Sexual Health (SASH) provides a Web site reference section where interested men can search for the names of sex addiction counselors in specific locations. The Web site is http://www.sash.net/.

The American Association of Pastoral Counselors also provides a geographic reference service. Note that not all pastoral counselors are trained to provide sexual addiction counseling. The Web site is: http://www.aapc.org/.

When the words sexual addiction counseling were entered into Google's search engine, more than a million hits were returned. Modify your search to sex addiction counselor followed by your city and state.

When searching for a counselor it is critical to find a competent person with whom you are comfortable. Ask if the counselor provides a consultation session. If so, in the session talk about the counseling methods the counselor uses. During that time you can assess your compatibility with the counselor.

Twelve Step programs

The following is an inventory of the major Twelve Step and related programs that are available to those who desire recovery from sexual addiction. The list contains the name, link to an internet Web page, and a brief description of the purpose of each organization. This book endorses Twelve Step programs but does not endorse a specific Twelve Step program. It is for you to decide which Twelve Step program best fits your needs. You may wish to try more than one program.

Twelve Step programs for the spouse or significant other

Codependents of Sexual Addiction (COSA)

The Web site is http://www.cosa-recovery.org/.

> Codependents of Sexual Addiction (COSA) is a recovery program for men and women whose lives have been affected by compulsive sexual behavior. In COSA, we find hope whether or not there is a sexually addicted person currently in our lives. With the humble act of reaching out, we begin the process of recovery.

> The COSA recovery program has been adapted from the Twelve Steps and Twelve Traditions of Alcoholics Anonymous and Al-Anon. It is a program for our spiritual development, no matter what our religious beliefs. As we meet to share our experience, strength and hope while working the twelve steps, we grow stronger in spirit. We begin to lead our lives more serenely and in deeper fulfillment, little by little, one day at a time. Only in this way can we be of help to others.

> COSA is open to anyone whose life has been affected by compulsive sexual behavior. Although there are no dues or fees for membership, most groups pass a basket for contributions since COSA is entirely self-supporting and declines outside donations.

S-Anon Family Groups

The Web site is http://www.sanon.org/.

> The S-Anon Family Groups are a fellowship of the relatives and friends of sexually addicted people who share their experience, strength and hope in order to solve their common problems. Our program of recovery is adapted from Alcoholics Anonymous and is based on the Twelve Steps and the Twelve Traditions of Alcoholics Anonymous. S-Anon's Twelve Concepts of Service provide guidance in serving each other in our business matters. There are no dues or fees for S-Anon membership; we are self-supporting through our own contributions.

> S-Anon is not allied with any sect, denomination, politics, organization or institution; it does not wish to engage in any controversy; nor does it endorse or oppose any causes. Our primary purpose is to recover from the effects upon us of another person's sexaholism and to help the families and friends of sexaholics. We do this by applying the Twelve Steps of S-Anon to our lives and by welcoming and giving comfort to families of sexaholics.

Twelve Step programs for the addict

Christians in Recovery

The Web site is http://christians-in-recovery.org/wp/

> Christians in Recovery (CIR) is a group of recovering Christians dedicated to mutual sharing of faith, strength and hope as we live each day in recovery. We work to regain and maintain balance and order in our lives through active discussion of the 12 Steps, the Bible, and experiences in our own recovery from abuse, family dysfunction, depression, anxiety, grief, relationships and/ or addictions of alcohol, drugs, food, pornography, sexual addiction, etc.

Sex Addicts Anonymous

The Web site is http://www.sexaa.org/.

> Sex Addicts Anonymous is a fellowship of men and women who share their experience, strength and hope with each other so they may overcome their sexual addiction and help others recover from sexual addiction and dependency. Membership is open to all who share a desire to stop addictive sexual behavior. There is no other requirement.

> Our common goals are to become sexually healthy and to help other sex addicts achieve freedom from compulsive sexual behavior. SAA is supported through voluntary contributions from members. We are not affiliated with any other Twelve-Step programs, nor are we a part of any other organization. We do not support, endorse, or oppose outside causes or issues.

> Sex Addicts Anonymous is a spiritual program based on the principles and traditions of Alcoholics Anonymous. We are grateful to A.A. for this gift which makes our recovery possible.

Sexaholics Anonymous (SA)

The Web site is http://www.sa.org/.

> Sexaholics Anonymous is a fellowship of men and women who share their experience, strength, and hope with each other that they may solve their common problem and help others to recover.

> The only requirement for membership is a desire to stop lusting and become sexually sober. There are no dues or fees for SA membership; we are self-supporting through our own contributions.

SA is not allied with any sect, denomination, politics, organization, or institution; does not wish to engage in any controversy; neither endorses nor opposes any causes.

Our primary purpose is to stay sexually sober and help others to achieve sexual sobriety. Sexaholics Anonymous is a recovery program based on the principles of Alcoholics Anonymous and received permission from AA to use its Twelve Steps and Twelve Traditions in 1979.

Sexual Compulsives Anonymous (SCA)

The Web site is http://www.sca-recovery.org/.

> Sexual Compulsives Anonymous is a fellowship of men and women who share their experience, strength and hope with each other, that they may solve their common problem and help others to recover from sexual compulsion.
>
> SCA is a Twelve Step fellowship, inclusive of all sexual orientations, open to anyone with a desire to recover from sexual compulsion. We are not group therapy, but a spiritual program that provides a safe environment for working on problems of sexual addiction and sexual sobriety.
>
> We believe we are not meant to repress our God-given sexuality, but to learn how to express it in ways that will not make unreasonable demands on our time and energy, place us in legal jeopardy, or endanger our mental, physical or spiritual health. Members are encouraged to develop a sexual recovery plan, defining sexual sobriety for themselves.
>
> There are no requirements for admission to our meetings: anyone having difficulties with sexual compulsion is welcome. The only requirement for membership is a desire to stop having compulsive sex. There are no dues or fees for SCA membership; we are self-supporting through our own contributions. SCA is not allied with any sect, denomination, politics, organization, or institution; does not wish to engage in any controversy; neither endorses nor opposes any causes.
>
> Our primary purpose is to stay sexually sober and to help others to achieve sexual sobriety.

Sex and Love Addicts Anonymous (SLAA)

The Web site is http://www.slaafws.org/.

Sex and Love Addicts Anonymous is a Twelve Step—Twelve Tradition oriented fellowship based on the model pioneered by Alcoholics Anonymous.

One of the resources we draw on is our willingness to stop acting out in our own personal bottom line addictive behavior on a daily basis. In addition, members reach out to others in the fellowship, practice the Twelve Steps and Twelve Traditions of S.L.A.A. and seek a relationship with a higher power to counter the destructive consequences of one or more addictive behaviors related to sex addiction, love addiction, dependency on romantic attachments, emotional dependency, and sexual, social and emotional anorexia.

We find a common denominator in our obsessive, compulsive patterns which renders any personal differences of sexual or gender orientation irrelevant.

Sexual Recovery Anonymous (SRA)

The Web site is http://www.sexualrecovery.org/.

> Sexual Recovery Anonymous (SRA) is a fellowship of men and women who share their experience, strength and hope with each other that they may solve their common problem and help others to recover.

> The only requirement for membership is a desire to stop compulsive sexual behavior. There are no dues or fees for SRA membership; we are self-supporting through our own contributions. SRA is not allied with any sect, denomination, politics, organization, or institution; does not wish to engage in any controversy; neither endorses nor opposes any causes.

> Our primary purpose is to stay sexually sober and help others achieve sobriety. Sobriety is the release from all compulsive and destructive sexual behaviors. We have found through our experience that sobriety includes freedom from masturbation and sex outside a mutually committed relationship.

> We believe that spirituality and self-love are antidotes to the addiction. We are walking towards a healthy sexuality.

Survivors of Incest Anonymous

The Web site is http://www.siawso.org/.

> Survivors of Incest Anonymous (SIA) is a self-help group of women and men, 18 years or older, who are guided by a set of 12 Suggested Steps and 12 Traditions, along with some slogans and the Serenity Prayer. There are no dues or fees. Everything that is said here, in the group meeting or member to member, must be held in strict confidence. We do not have any professional therapist working in our group. SIA is not a replacement for therapy or any other professional service when needed. The only requirement for membership is that you are a victim of child sexual abuse, and you are not abusing any child. We define incest very broadly as a sexual experience by a family member or

by an extended family member that damaged the child. "Extended family" may include an aunt, uncle, in-law, step-parent, cousin, friend of the family, teacher, coach, another child, clergy or anyone that you were led to trust. We believe we were affected by the abuse whether it occurred once or many times since the damage is incurred immediately.

We learn in SIA not to deny, that we did not imagine the incest, nor was it our fault in any way. The abuser will go to any length to shift the responsibility to the defenseless child, often accusing the child of being seductive. We had healthy, natural needs for love, attention and acceptance, and we often paid high prices to get those needs met, but we did not seduce our abuser. Physical coercion is rarely necessary with a child since the child is already intimidated. The more gentle the assault, the more guilt the victim inappropriately carries. We also learn not to accept any responsibility for the assaults even if these occurred over a prolonged period of time. Some of us are still being sexually assaulted.

In SIA we share our experiences and common feelings. We realize that we thought we had to protect our caretakers from this horrible secret, as if they were not participants. We felt alienated from the non-abusive family members. Often, greater anger is directed toward them since it is safer to get angry at people we perceive to be powerless. We became caretakers in order to maintain an image of a nurturing family. Our feelings of betrayal by our families are immeasurable. We need to mourn the death of the ideal family that many of us created in our own imaginations.

In dealing with this pain, it feels as if we are pulling the scab off a wound that never healed properly, AND IT HURTS. However, it is easier to cry when we have friends who are not afraid of our tears. We CAN be comforted—that is why we are here. Our pain is no longer in vain. We will never forget, but we can, in time, end the regretting that accompanies destructive remembering. We can learn, One Day at a Time, that we are incest SURVIVORS, rather than incest victims.

Incest Survivors Anonymous (ISA)

The Web site is http://www.lafn.org/medical/isa/home.html.

Incest Survivors Anonymous (ISA) is:
A spiritual program.
A Twelve Step and Twelve Tradition program.
For incest survivors and prosurvivors. Prosurvivor is someone who loves, believes, and supports the survivor in their recovery from incest, such as a family member, spouse, friend.
An anonymous fellowship.
Self-help, peer-help.

Unconditional love.
For men, women, teens.

Recovering Couples Anonymous (RCA)

The Web site is http://www.recovering-couples.org/.

Recovering Couples Anonymous (RCA) is a 12-Step Fellowship founded in the Autumn of 1988. There are groups throughout the United States, as well as worldwide. Although there is no organizational affiliation with Alcoholics Anonymous, The 12 Steps, 12 Traditions and Principles are adapted from AA.

The primary purpose of RCA is to help couples find freedom from dysfunctional patterns in relationships. By using the tools of the program, we take individual responsibility for the well-being of the relationship, build new joy, and find intimacy with each other.

We are couples committed to restoring healthy communication, caring and greater intimacy to our relationships. We suffer from many addictions and co-addictions; some identified and some not, some treated and some not. We also come from different levels of brokenness. Many of us have been separated or near divorce. Some of us are new in our relationships and seek to build intimacy as we grow together as couples.

References

American Psychiatric Association. (2000). Diagnostic and Statistical Manual of Mental Disorders (4th ed, Text Revision). Washington, DC: American Psychiatric Association.

Arterburn, S., Stoeker, F., & Yorkey, M. (2000). Every Man's Battle: Winning the War on Sexual Temptation One Victory at a Time. Colorado Springs, CO: WaterBrook Press.

Beattie, M (1992). Codependent No More: How to Stop Controlling Others and Start Caring for Yourself. Center City, Mn: Hazelden Publishing; 2nd ed.

Becker, P (2010). In Search of Recovery: A Christian Man's Guide. Carefree, AZ: Gentle Path Press.

Becker, P (2010) In Search of Recovery Workbook: A Christian Man's Guide. Carefree, AZ: Gentle Path Press.

Bradshaw, J. (1988). Bradshaw on: The Family. Deerfield Beach, FL: Health Communications.

Bradshaw, J. (2005). Healing the Shame That Binds You. Deerfield Beach, FL: Health Communications.

Broucek, F., (1991). Shame and the Self. New York, NY: Guilford Press.

Carnes, P. (1983). Out of the Shadows: Understanding Sexual Addiction. Minneapolis, MN: CompCare Publications.

Carnes, P. (1994). Out of the Shadows: Understanding Sexual Addiction. Center City, MN: Hazelden Publishing, 2nd ed.

Carnes P. (1989). Contrary To Love: Helping the Sexual Addict. Minneapolis, MN: CompCare Publications.

Carnes P. (1991). Don't Call it Love: Recovering From Sexual Addiction. New York: Bantam.

Carnes, P. (2001). Facing the Shadow: Starting Sexual and Relationship Recovery.

Paul Becker, LPC

Wickenburg, AZ: Gentle Path Press.

Covenant Eyes (Last retrieved January 28, 2012.) http://www.covenanteyes.com/

Family Safe Media. (Retrieved January 25, 2012). http://www.familysafemedia.com/pornography_statistics.html

Ferree, M. (Retrieved January 28, 2012) http://bethesdaworkshops.org/staff/marnie-c-ferree/

Galifianakis, Z (2011). Cartoon, Washington Post. Washington DC

Holy Bible, New International Version (NIV)

Laaser, D. (Retrieved January 28, 2012.). http://www.faithandtrueministries.com/about/bios-pics/

Laaser, M. (Retrieved January 28, 2012.). http://www.nationalcoalitition.org/imagges/Kansas/%20City/MARK%20ROBERT%20LASSER%20Bio.pdf

Melody, P, Miller, A. W., & Miller, J. K. (1989). Facing Codependence: What It Is, Where It Comes from, How It Sabotages Our Lives. New York, NY: Harper & Row; 1st ed.

Morrison, K. (February 24, 2004) Battling Sexual Addiction. Dateline: MSNBC Interactive News, LCC. Last retrieved January 28, 2012. http://www.msnbc.msn.com/id/4302347/ns/dateline_nbc/t/battling-sexual-addiction/

Maltz W. (2001). The Sexual Healing Journey: A Guide for Survivors of Sexual Abuse. New York, NY: Quill

Panos, A. (No date). Healing from Shame with Traumatic Events. Last retrieved January 28, 2012. http://www.giftfromwithin.org/html/healing.html

Schneider, J., Corley, M., & Irons, R.(1998). Surviving Disclosure of Infidelity: Results of an International Survey of 164 Recovering Sex Addicts and Partners. Sexual Addiction & Compulsivity, 5,3, 189-217

Sex Addicts Anonymous (SAA). (Retrieved 2009). http://www.sexaa.org/addict.htm

Recidivism in Virginia. (2001). Tracking the 1997 release cohort. Virginia Department of Corrections. Last retrieved January 28, 2012. http://www.vadoc.virginia.gov/about/facts/research/recidivism/recidivism01.doc

Recidivism in Virginia. (2003). Tracking the 1998 release cohort. Virginia Department of Corrections. Last retrieved January 28, 2012. http://www.vadoc.virginia.gov/about/facts/research/recidivism/recidivism03.doc

Recidivism in Virginia. (2005). <u>Tracking the 1999 release cohort</u>. Virginia Department of Corrections. Last retrieved January 28, 2012. http://www.vadoc.state.va.us/about/facts/ research/recidivism/recidivism05.doc

US Department of Justice (2003). <u>Recidivism of Sex Offenders Released from Prison in 1994.</u> Last retrieved January 28, 2012. <u>http://bjs.ojp.usdoj.gov/content/pub/pdf/rpr94.pdf</u>

Willingham, R. (1999) <u>Breaking Free:Understanding Sexual Addiction & the Healing Power of Jesus</u>. Downers Grove, Il: InterVarsity Press.